"I have worked with Dr. McKnight for nearly 12 years. He is a colleague who is respected among his peers as a progressive thinker and committed to preventive medicine. This book is a reflection of his uniquely, open-minded, insightful approach. I use this water at home for the health benefits outlined in this book. As a supporter of the green movement I also use ionized water because it is environmentally responsible. Water is the key to all life, now we are finding it is the key to all health."

---Galen Durose, Jr, M.D. (Family Medicine)

"After practicing critical care medicine for over 20 years and surviving breast cancer, I only wished I had learned about the role of ionized water in cellular healing years ago. I have invested in a unit and highly recommend to my medical colleagues that they study the contents of this book with an open mind. It is not a stretch for me to anticipate the day when ionizers become standard equipment in intensive care units."

---Jennifer Ney, D.O. (Pulmonary & Critical Care Medicine)

"Dr. McKnight has clearly done his research and made a scientifically sound argument for the benefits of ionized water, while maintaining perspective on the entire portrait of health. I am a believer who recommends the water to my patients."

---Colin Chan, M.D. (Family Medicine)

"Dr. McKnight has written a book that is well-documented and scientifically grounded. As a scientist trained to think critically and logically, this book passes the test."

---Jean Engohang-Ndong, Ph.D. (Microbiologist)

D0019100

1

"As one who believes in sound nutritional practices for the health of the eye, this piece has opened my eyes to one of the most powerful, preventive tools I have ever come across. Well done, Dr. McKnight."

---Scott Keating, OD (Optometrist)

"This is a fascinating concept about ionized water, which makes perfectly good sense. I have come across this book for the first time and hope to start drinking this water myself and with my family. Thank you, Dr. McKnight, for all your time and energy to enlighten me and others."

---Mohammad Jan, M.D. (Cardiologist)

"After reading this book I have gained new insights that are applicable to my practice. As a Board Certified Wound Care Specialist and director of a wound care center, I feel ionized water has the potential to markedly improve the delivery of healthcare around the globe."

---Jon Oliverio, DPM/CWS (Podiatrist/Wound Care Specialist)

"This book embraces the holistic approach to medicine that my profession stands for. I whole-heartedly recommend this book to my colleagues and patients."

---Mike Jakubowski, D.C.

CONFESSIONS OF A SKEPTICAL PHYSICIAN

by TIM McKNIGHT M.D.

CONTENTS:

Disclaimer

The information in this book is being presented to help you understand the topics being discussed. It is not intended as a substitute for any treatment that may have been recommended by your doctor or any medications that have been prescribed for you.

If you suspect that you have any medical problems, we urge you to seek competent medical advice and care from health care professionals you can actually sit with and review your specific symptoms, history, needs and desires.

The best medical care is individual. Appropriate treatment is on a case-by-case basis. Everyone deserves the best medical care possible. We hope you learn from the information in this book and use it in your interactions with your healthcare providers.

Purpose

This book was written to help explain why anyone interested in optimizing their health should seriously consider drinking ionized water. What I originally dismissed as "snake oil hype" has developed into a healthy respect and deep interest in the complex nature of water. In 2003 Dr. Peter Agre and Dr. Roderick MacKinnon received the Nobel Prize in chemistry for the description of Water Channels that are present in every cell through which only water can pass. This milestone achievement has opened up entirely new research areas in biochemistry and biology. The work of Dr. Gerald Pollock from the University of Washington has provided fascinating evidence that water exists as a "liquid crystal" on surface interfaces and surrounding cellular components.[1] What was once considered a simple molecule is now attracting the attention of leading researchers who are discovering the complex and biologically significant applications of water, yes water, which is contained in every cell in our bodies.

As a result of my studies on this topic, it has become clear to me that science and medicine have long overlooked the complex role of water in biological systems. While I may not succeed at persuading you to agree with all of my conclusions, I sincerely hope that this book will at least stimulate you to ask questions and do your own research, like I continue to do, as my fascination with, and respect for water continues to grow.

My intent is to convince EVERYONE, especially healthcare professionals, that health is a matter of putting the body in a state of equilibrium and balance, and that ionized water offers one of the most simple, effective and cost-saving ways to help achieve this balance. I have tried to explain the basic chemistry for the novice and also included abstracts at the end of the book for the scientifically minded, to facilitate digging deeper.

I hope you read this book critically and challenge much of what is written. I am okay with that approach; in fact, I encourage you to investigate as I did, and to stay open minded during the process.

Statistics indicate that over two-thirds of the US population is overweight. We're living in a super sized, soft drink, fast food society. The only running most people do is back to the refrigerator. The only time most people drink water, is to swallow their prescription medicine. Something needs to change.

This book is dedicated to every patient who has been misinformed, or thinks that healing is achieved only through medication. THAT THEORY IS WRONG! Healing is a built-in mechanism within each of us. We can heal when we nurture, nourish, exercise, rest and love our bodies. Before plants or animals could exist, water had to be present. Science maintains that life originated in water. This seems logical since life involves biochemical reactions. We are over 70% water. Water is the most important molecule in the universe!

My Background

For as long as I can remember I wanted to be a doctor. When I was a teenager I wanted to combine my interest in portrait drawing with surgery and become a plastic surgeon. As an athlete, my interests expanded to include nutrition and exercise physiology. I was further influenced by my mother who ran several weight loss franchises and my father who taught high school biology and coached at every level of sports from amateur to high school, collegiate and even at the Olympic level.

I have always asked questions. Why does the body respond to this diet or that training protocol? What role does the mind play in health and healing? What is the root cause of chronic disease? Why does a particular treatment work on one person but not another?

In 1978 I began my undergraduate studies, majoring in pre-med. From 1979 to 1981 I took a break from my studies to proclaim my religious convictions in Austria. At the young age of nineteen I learned to listen to others before I spoke, respect those who had different belief systems from mine, and communicate my beliefs as clearly and respectfully as I could. I learned to be tolerant of others, sensitive to human emotion, and to be more in tune with what I was about.

Upon returning from Austria I continued my studies at Brigham Young University. At the age of 21 I was determined to complete my pre-medical studies in preparation for medical school. After a mediocre freshman year, the pre-med advisor convinced me that my 3.0 GPA would mathematically nullify my chances for medical school admission. Because I yielded my belief system to his, and not my own, I changed my goals and my major to Food Science and Nutrition. That one decision, based upon someone else's opinion, took me on an eight-year diversion through graduate school. It was also the last time I would allow someone else to write my story. Four years later, in 1985, BS degree in hand, I was enrolled in the doctorate program at Ohio State University.

Nutritional Training

For the next eight years I pursued my doctorate degree and worked fulltime as the department's laboratory technician in order to provide for my wife and young children. In this capacity I assisted fellow grad students with their PhD and master's research, ran and maintained laboratory equipment, performed my own doctoral research, and completed all the written and oral examinations to meet the requirements for my PhD in Human Nutrition.

Three years into this process I decided I wanted to rewrite my story and apply nutritional sciences as a physician, not as a scientist. I had done well in my coursework and thoroughly enjoyed and was fascinated by nutritional biochemistry and exercise physiology. After being accepted into the College of Medicine at Ohio State University, all I needed to do was complete a research project to meet the requirements for the doctorate degree. For the next two years I dedicated myself to two separate research projects that failed — for a number of reasons over which I had little control. My research focused on the metabolism of branched-chained amino acids and how the key regulatory enzyme of these essential amino acids was influenced by weight loss, exercise and trauma.

In the summer of 1992 I finally found a project that moved forward but I was running out of time. I had postponed my entry into medical school for two years to complete my research, but the College of Medicine was not willing to defer my entry another year. By the fall of 1993 I had completed nearly 60 percent of my research and I projected it would take six more months to complete the doctoral program. That August I also began medical school, while working part time for the Department of Surgery and taking care of my expanding family (now three children). Needless to say, my schedule was unmanageable, and as a result I made one of the hardest decisions of my life. In October of 1993 I withdrew from graduate school after eight years of sacrifice and study. I was only six months short of earning a PhD. I was exhausted and devastated, yet determined to move forward and apply my nutritional studies in a clinical setting.

My graduate studies taught me to be a critical thinker, to be skeptical of any health claim that was not backed by sound research, preferably double-blinded, random, placebo-controlled studies. In fact, many of my graduate courses required that I carefully review and critique research, looking for flaws in thought or design that could discredit the results. I learned about statistics and research terms like "random assignment," "p-values," "regression analysis," and "correlations." I learned that "statistically significant" does not always mean "clinically significant." I also learned about the "dark side" of science. I witnessed the manipulation and intimidation that can occur when large amounts of grant funding and tenure are on the line. Occasionally I saw statistics massaged to advance a project. I had more than one discussion with fellow grad students about these challenges. We felt caught in the middle of the pressure to get results and walk the thin line between ethics and objectivity.

I left the scientific world dismayed and cynical. However, I soon learned in medicine that scientific process and clinical studies, flawed as they sometimes are, is the only way to safely advance the science of medicine. Without the scientific method, healthcare would not be as advanced as it is today.

On the other hand, my graduate and medical school experiences taught me to ask, "Who stands to gain financially with the advancement of this treatment, this drug or this program?" In other words, who is asking the question and why? Clearly, both the question and the questioner can affect the answer.

Medical Training

I felt extremely fortunate to attend the Ohio State College of Medicine. It has a strong reputation of being one of the finest medical schools in the country, especially in preparing student-doctors for careers in primary care, like my chosen field of Family Medicine. Like all allopathic medical schools, the emphasis was not on disease prevention it was on disease identification, diagnosis and management. At the time, there was very little instruction on nutritional biochemistry — we had too much pharmacology to learn. As a medical student I soon sensed that my 13 years of undergraduate and graduate studies were of little clinical value. We were too busy cramming anatomy, embryology, histology, and patho-physiology into our brains.

After two years of classroom learning, medical schools typically send students to clinics and hospital wards to follow mentoring physicians. We learn to regurgitate medical information and try not to make any major mistakes in front of preceptors who have the power to fail us on their rotation. My clinical preceptors were for the most part exemplary, competent and compassionate. Nevertheless, I was graded on my clinical acumen to correctly diagnose and treat disease, NEVER on preventing or reversing it!

After graduating from medical school I was very fortunate to be accepted into one of the best Family

Medicine residency programs in the region — Grant Medical Center in Columbus, Ohio. It was a demanding training program but I really felt I was working with some of the best clinicians on the planet! As an intern I was on call every fifth night, meaning I got little sleep and spent many hours in the middle of the night in the emergency room or caring for critically ill patients in the intensive care unit. The end of each long shift was met with extreme fatigue but also an emotional high knowing we had actually kept critically ill patients alive by following protocols we had been taught. Three years of this kind of training brings a confidence in medical decision-making that is not present upon graduation from medical school. While I learned to manage disease and perform multiple invasive procedures in residency, I did not learn how to prevent disease other than with immunizations.

By the year 2000 I had completed three years of medical residency. At the age of 40, I was finally ready for my first job! Because I received a scholarship from the National Health Services Corp during my last three years of medical school, I was obligated to provide three years of service in a medically underserved community. I chose a small community hospital in northeastern Ohio.

My practice quickly grew and I began treating the common chronic diseases of high blood pressure, diabetes, elevated cholesterol, heart disease, acid reflux, obesity, gout, arthritis, etc., etc. I soon realized that a healthy lifestyle could reverse many of these diseases or at the very least reduce the

13

dependence of so many of my patients on numerous pharmaceuticals. Unfortunately, I was not able to educate them about proper diet, exercise and stress management during the 15-minute slot allotted to each patient.

In 2002 I attended a medical conference to learn how to develop a "Wellness Prescription" for my patients. As I sat through the entire week of lectures I realized that I already knew how to do this — simply apply the nutrition and exercise physiology principles I had learned in graduate school. When I returned from the course I committed myself to developing a program that would benefit my patients and anyone else who wanted to restore their health.

This program was launched in 2003. I offered it after my office hours, without personal compensation, because I believed my patients wanted to heal from, and not just manage, many of these chronic diseases. The format was a ten-week course that was primarily based on sound nutrition and exercise practices. Body weight, body fat, cholesterol levels, blood pressure and other measures were assessed at the beginning and end of the program. For want of a better name, the program was called, "Fit for Life." It was effective for those who followed the plan, but the $450 per person cost to administer the program was prohibitive. After three series of classes, the cost proved to be the death of the program.

I returned to my office frustrated that I was forced back into a medical model that paid me only to treat disease, not prevent it. I was not helping my patients get healthy and I was not happy. I became very disillusioned with the allopathic model of disease management and I felt I too was its victim. Fortunately, in 2005 the marketing director of the hospital, also a talented grant writer, remembered the positive impact of my initial program and submitted a grant application to the Health Resources and Service Administration's Office of Rural Health Policy. A year later we were awarded a $375,000 grant and I was appointed medical director of the program.

This funding allowed me to educate my patients and the community on healthy nutrition, exercise and stress management. At the conclusion of the original three-year grant, the community support and results were so favorable that a second grant, taking the same program into the worksite, was awarded. To date, $750,000 of grant funding has been awarded to my team and more than 1,200 adults have completed this 12-week series of classes. One hundred percent of participants have said they would recommend the program to their family and friends. I finally felt like I was making a difference and helping people heal from within.

My Introduction to Ionized Water

It was during one of the worksite
wellness classes that I was introduced
to ionized water. After one class,
Linda, who was a Fit for Life
participant, approached me and said,
"You really need to learn about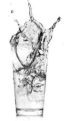
ionized water. I think you would be fascinated and
I think it would fit in with what you have been
telling our class." I asked a few questions for
clarification and thought to myself, "I don't have
time for this, it sounds like a scam." For the next
several weeks Linda would invite me to a
"demonstration meeting." I thought to myself,
"This is crazy, doesn't she understand that H_2O is
just H_2O? There is nothing more to it."

Linda's persistence was bordering on annoying. I
finally agreed to attend a meeting primarily to show
her the respect she had given to me and my
message. I was only slightly interested in this
concept and totally expected to poke holes in the
logic and chemistry of her "ionized water".

When the meeting began I sat smugly in my seat,
listening to the speaker, who was an acupuncturist.
I was thinking, "I am not falling for this nonsense. I
will not be tricked or persuaded by anything he
says." I was still confident in my position until I
saw the testing done on various liquids, including
many commonly consumed bottled water products.
When I saw the pH meter, I felt like I was back in
my research lab, my comfort zone. When the ORP

16

(Oxidation-Reduction Potential) meter was used, I was even more fascinated with the results I was seeing. I would have to learn more.

I read all the materials that were supplied, most of which were testimonials. These were not persuasive to me at all — anyone can give a testimonial. I needed facts. But I could not stop thinking about the results that objectively showed a distinct difference between ionized water and most other consumable fluids. My initial search on the Internet led me to articles warning of ionized water "scams" but these claims also lacked scientific substance and were based on personal opinion, so I discarded those criticisms.

In the weeks that followed, Linda loaned us one of her ionizers and we experimented with it on ourselves and on our children. My health was good but I noted more energy, clearer thinking and faster recovery from strenuous exercise. My teenage son stopped experiencing migraine headaches when he drank it and commented on the improvement in his acne and his stamina on the basketball court. My youngest daughter used the water to help detangle her hair and it seemed to work just as well as the conditioners she was using.

The most impressive observation I made was with my wife, Karen. She had injured her shoulder in a fall two years prior and subsequently developed a frozen shoulder that failed to respond to conventional physical therapy, chiropractic manipulation or massage therapy. Having successfully rehabilitated through this condition myself and confident in my clinical skills to help her, I was disappointed that she was so disabled and had failed therapies that usually work. I suggested she submit to orthopedic manipulation of the adhesions under anesthesia. Her sister suggested she drink more ionized water as a therapeutic trial. Karen decided she had nothing to lose.

She was unable to lift her arm to brush her hair and was waking at night, crying with pain. I left for work that morning and through the course of the day she drank over a gallon of freshly made ionized water. To my utter surprise, that evening when I returned home, she lifted her arm above her head and demonstrated for me her improved, pain-free range of motion that was now nearly 90% of normal! I was completely amazed! I had no idea how or why this occurred but I knew the water had done something to restore her motion. The change has been permanent. I would not have believed it without seeing it!

As I witnessed these experiences firsthand and listened to the stories of other users of the water I began to soften my attitude and become more intrigued. Still, my clinical, scientific mind was telling me, "Don't talk to your colleagues or patients about this, they'll think you're crazy." I knew these observations were nothing more than testimonials. Could they be placebo effects? Was there any science behind this?

I became a student of ionization and what the electrolysis process did to alter water's chemistry. I also began finding scientific evidence supporting many of the health claims I was hearing about and starting to see in patients who were using the water faithfully. I was especially reassured when I came across published research that described the ability of ionized water to neutralize the oxidative damage caused by free radicals.

In addition to utilizing standard medical wisdom and published research, one of my personal requirements when treating disease is that the treatments must agree with current knowledge of biochemistry, physiology, and anatomy. Everything I have learned about ionized water is supported by the basic principles of these disciplines.

Ionized water supports the body's natural healing process; it does not *directly* heal anything. It is a great supporter of wellness but cannot be expected to support a healing biochemistry when the individual is repeatedly exposed to the heavy oxidative burdens of cigarettes, excess alcohol, drug use, extreme emotional stress, or diets contaminated by high amounts of high fructose corn syrup, hydrogenated fats, pesticide-laden produce, etc. Common sense and sound chemistry still must prevail and I am confident it does with regards to the benefits of ionized water.

Initially I was reluctant to suggest the use of ionized water to my patients. What if they bought an ionizer and noticed nothing favorable? What about my reputation? I did not want to risk violating their trust in me as their physician. I also had to be true to the Hippocratic oath and my commitment to "do no harm." However, as I began seeing results in my family and myself AND as I found mounting research publications supporting the use of ionized water, I began to feel I could not withhold what I was learning from patients whom I felt might benefit from using it.

The Root Cause of Chronic Disease

The root cause of disease is stress. *Stress is defined as a straining force, an imbalance of forces.* Stress is a form of opposition that stimulates adaptation, growth and development in any life form exposed to it. Stress is only "bad" when it is excessive, unbalanced and unchecked.

The stress of pressure turns graphite into diamonds. The stress of sunlight is captured by chlorophyll in plants and converted into an energy form (glucose) that feeds the growth of the plant. The stress of the birthing process gives rise to new life. It was stress that formed the Grand Canyon, Niagara Falls and the Hawaiian Islands. Stress on muscles force them to grow in response to the opposition they encounter. Stress is a necessary stimulus for life. It is a catalyst for beauty and growth. However, when stress exceeds our limits to contain and manage it, disharmony and imbalance result.

In living organisms, unchecked, unbalanced stress is the stimulus for disease. I will present three of the most common types that I have seen and managed as a physician — oxidative stress, acidic stress and hydration stress. All forms need to be understood and managed if healing is to occur. The more accumulative stress we experience in these three categories, the more diseased our cells become and the more effort is needed to balance the body so that real healing can occur.

Oxidative Stress

Oxidative stress is the root cause of chronic disease. It is also believed to be responsible for the aging process.[2] In simple terms *oxidative stress is the chemical process of stealing electrons.* It is a natural and predictable part of day-to-day cellular activity.

The messenger of oxidative stress is a *free radical.* A free radical is a one of the simplest chemical structures. To understand the free radical requires an understanding of the atomic nature of matter.

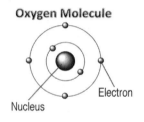

Oxygen Molecule

Nucleus

Electron

All atoms (elements) are single units compromised of a nucleus, which is made up of a specific number of neutrons and positively charged protons. Surrounding this nucleus is an energy cloud comprised of negatively charged particles called electrons. Electrons are located in specific orbits or "shells" around the nucleus of the atom. *The key concept that must be appreciated to understand oxidative stress is that the atom is stable when electrons are paired with other electrons.* But under conditions of oxidative stress, electrons can become separated from their partner. A single, unpaired electron creates an unbalanced, stressful state. **This is the definition of a free radical — an unpaired,**

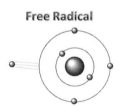

Free Radical

unstable electron. When electrons are pulled away from their partner, this is oxidative stress!

In an effort to find stability, free radicals "steal" an electron from a neighboring atom. This satisfies the original atom's need for stability and balance but creates a free radical in the second atom because it loses its paired electrical state. This begins a cascade of events, the cellular equivalent of a dangerous nuclear reaction. The process of stealing electrons propagates rapidly from atom to atom, often until a vulnerable endpoint is reached when irreversible damage is done to key cellular components — proteins (both inside the cell and the receptors on the cell membranes), lipids (fatty acids found inside the cell and in the cellular membrane) or nucleic acid (i.e., DNA or RNA).

FREE RADICALS IN THE HUMAN BODY

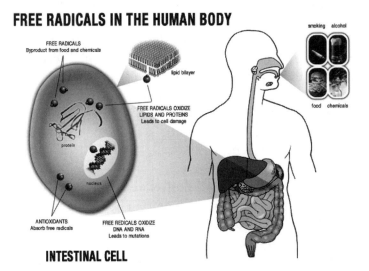

INTESTINAL CELL

Even though the life of a free radical is estimated to be only a millionth of a second, this is long enough to be destructive to cellular structures.

Some of the most common cellular free radicals are hydroxyl radical (-OH), singlet oxygen ($^1O_2$), superoxide anion radical (-O_2), and hydrogen peroxide (H_2O_2). Note that these free radicals all contain oxygen, the very atom required for life. Oxygen is nature's oxymoron — it is required for life but too much can disrupt it. In fact, the immune system uses byproducts of oxygen metabolism (-OH, -O_2, H_2O_2) to generate free radicals that destroy microbes (bacteria, viruses, fungi, parasites) that threaten the host.

The blood, via the RBC, is the vehicle that carries oxygen to every cell in the body. Oxygen is literally "the breath of life." The Bible states in Leviticus 17:11, "For the life of the flesh is in the blood." While for most Christians this is a reference to eternal life and the blood of Christ, a more literal application regarding life itself is also true. Without the oxygen carried in blood there would be no life. Limit oxygen and you compromise the healing of tissues. Withdraw it and death is guaranteed.

Free radicals are continually generated through normal metabolic processes. The oxygen we breathe is used to combust the fuels of our body, primarily fatty acids, glucose, and at times amino acids from protein. During this combustion process free radicals are generated. This is a natural process.

Fortunately, every cell is equipped with numerous powerful antioxidants and enzyme systems that neutralize free radicals by donating an available free electron. When we eat nature's foods we replenish both the antioxidants and the enzyme systems that are composed of key minerals (i.e., selenium, zinc, copper, manganese, etc.) that further neutralize oxidative stress and keep it in check. However, when we choose lifestyles that invite more oxidative stress than we can balance through the process of *reduction,* (electron donation) oxidative stress results and disease knocks on the door.

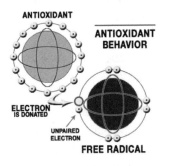

The role of tissue antioxidants is so critical that key electron donors are strategically placed in and around the cell to neutralize the oxidative threat of free radical destruction. For example, Vitamin E, a fat-soluble molecule is the primary guardian against free radical attack to the lipid-core of cell membranes. Inside the cell Vitamin C and Glutathione contribute to protect the cytoplasm from oxidative stress. The mitochondria of the cell is a uniquely stressed site because it is here that oxygen is converted into an energy form. This requires ample supplies of the very capable, protein anti-oxidant, CoEnzymeQ10. Unfortunately, the use of statin drugs for cholesterol management often depletes this anti-oxidant leading to fatigue, muscle aches, joint pain, and comprised muscle function. Finally, the fluids around cells are protected by the water-soluble vitamin C (ascorbic acid). These four anti-oxidants are only a partial list of key body anti-oxidants. Several enzyme systems also exist.

An even more important clue concerning the vital role of anti-oxidants in the body is underscored by the fact that these molecules often regenerate each other to protect themselves from becoming free radicals after donating their spare electrons. For example, Vitamin C can regenerate Vitamin E. Beta-carotene is regenerated from Vitamin C, Vitamin E, and selenium. Vitamin C is regenerated by alpha-lipoic acid and procyanthocyanidins.

Despite these extremely efficient and powerful natural defenses against oxidative stress, two key processes can reduce our capacity to maintain this balance — inadequate nutritional protection and overwhelming exposure to free radicals. While the foods we eat and the quality of the water we drink may support our inherent protective systems, external exposures to harmful chemicals often tip the scales away from balance and towards oxidative stress.

One of the most toxic, destructive sources of oxidative stress via free radicals is *tobacco*.[3,4] Cigarette smoking is a physician's nightmare. It is strongly associated with heart disease, numerous cancers, emphysema and impaired wound healing due to poor blood circulation. Tobacco use is oxidative stress on steroids!

Another highly toxic, free radical-creating poison is *alcohol*. It may well be the most commonly abused drug in the world. It attacks the human liver. Alcohol is absorbed directly from the stomach and carried by venous blood to the liver. The liver gets the first look at everything we eat and drink. It is a clearinghouse for toxins. It tries to destroy or neutralize harmful compounds before they can enter the general circulation and gain access to every cell in the body. Repeated insults from alcohol exerts stress on the antioxidant systems within this vital organ, leading to reversible, and then later irreversible oxidative damage, before this organ eventually fails. Alcohol also damages the esophageal and stomach linings through direct tissue oxidative stress, leaving both tissues vulnerable to cancer and to life-threatening ulcers and bleeding.

Radiant energy can also be excessive and create a burden beyond the body's antioxidant defense systems. Ultraviolet light, especially UVB rays from repeated and prolonged sun exposure, can disrupt the protein collagen, which provides structural support to the skin. Over time, sunbathers tend to develop leathery, wrinkly skin, signs of oxidative stress. Not surprisingly, alcohol and tobacco use also age the skin, affecting collagen by the same mechanism.

Nature's pure, unadulterated foods were created for us. Most of these foods are slightly alkaline and rich in antioxidants. This is how the Creator of the universe intended it to be. It is for our benefit. Every attempt by man to improve or modify the plants that nourish us has failed miserably and resulted in *foods with inferior nutritional value*. For example, in the production of enriched flours, whole grains are modified and refined as part of the milling process and in so doing the key antioxidant nutrients are stripped from these whole grains. By the middle of the 20th century this process resulted in many common nutritional deficiencies in humans. It took an act of congress (The Enrichment Act of 1942) to pass a law mandating that all processed flours must be enriched with four key, essential nutrients. The truth is that even "enriched" flour is lacking many other trace elements, vitamins and minerals removed during the milling process.

This is not nature's way; it is man's way. The result has been a significant loss of free radical-neutralizing compounds from foods inherently designed to protect us. In fact, a recent study has shown that high sugar diets have a direct effect on free radical formation and oxidative stress.[5,6] Even *eating a diet in excess of caloric needs* can cause oxidative stress![7] Furthermore, cooking or frying with *hydrogenated fats* is a recipe for free radical synthesis! It is one of the most dangerous nutritional practices of our day! Yet, this is the practice of nearly every fast food restaurant in the world. What are we thinking?

Acidic Stress

Acidic Stress is a precursor to oxidative stress. By definition, acidic stress is the result of chronic acid exposure, primarily from diets high in sugars, animal protein (especially red meat and dairy products), emotional stress, physical stress (via lactic acid buildup) or elimination problems such as kidney failure.

The body goes to extreme measures to maintain a slightly alkaline pH in most tissues. For example, blood, the lifeline of the body, has an optimal pH of 7.35 – 7.45. Three primary buffering systems exist to help maintain this narrow pH window, underscoring the critical nature of pH in optimal physiology. The most powerful and rapid buffering system is the lungs. The faster we breathe the more acidic carbon dioxide we exhale, taking us back towards neutrality. Heavy breathing with exercise is a prime example of this quick and efficient mechanism of buffering the blood.

The kidneys are the second major buffering system. Urine with a mean pH of 6.0 is nearly 15 times as acidic as blood because its role is to eliminate much of the acidic buildup that occurs within the body as a result of metabolism and exercise. When blood becomes overly acidic, the kidneys can reabsorb alkaline bicarbonate and excrete acidic hydrogen ions. This is a slower process that can take hours to days to fully buffer the blood but this system can do so with extreme precision, especially when the lungs are damaged because of health issues like chronic obstructive pulmonary disease (COPD).

The final means of achieving a slightly alkaline state is through chemical buffers, either inside or outside of cells. Inside the cell three quarters of all chemical buffers are proteins. Outside the cells the largest buffering pool in the body is found in the bones in the form of calcium carbonate and calcium phosphate. Unfortunately, repeated acidic assaults on the body in the form of extremely acidic soft drinks, diets high in sugars, animal proteins (i.e., meats and dairy products) and processed foods but low in plant foods (i.e., vegetables, legumes, beans, nuts, seeds, etc.) result in the release of calcium carbonate from the bones to buffer this acidic burden at the expense of calcium bone stores, enhancing the development of osteoporosis and possibly kidney stones.

Ninety-nine percent of the calcium is in the bones. It provides a huge reservoir upon which the body can draw to neutralize chronic states of acidosis. Bones can take up acid in exchange for calcium, sodium and potassium (ionic exchange) or release the buffers of bicarbonate.

Bone is a very large buffering system. Green and Kleeman reported that 80 percent of total body carbonate is in the hydration shell, the water surrounding bone.[8] In other words, an alkaline solution is believed to surround bone, underscoring the critical nature of protecting bone from acidic insults.

30

In states of chronic acidity the major buffering mechanism by far is release of calcium carbonate from the bones. The mechanism by which this dissolution of bone crystal occurs involves two processes:

- Direct chemical breakdown of bone crystals in response to acid overload
- Bone cell destruction by the bone dissolving cells, the osteoclast

The average American diet, which is high in protein and low in fruits and vegetables, can generate a significant amount of acid daily (100 mEq) mainly in the form of phosphate and sulfate.[9] Such a diet raises the acid burden and the need for alkaline-rich water. By drinking this water we may preserve bone minerals and limit the release of calcium into the blood, thus lowering the risk of developing both kidney stones and gout.

There are several other diseases that thrive in acidic states. *Gastroesophageal Reflux Disease* (GERD) is perhaps the most common. In addition to the acidic diets mentioned above, other risk factors for GERD include the use of caffeine, tobacco and alcohol. These chemicals prevent a muscle at the end of the esophagus (the lower esophageal sphincter) from tightly closing after food enters the stomach, resulting in acid splashing out of the stomach and up into the esophagus.

Abdominal obesity is another common cause of GERD. In obesity the enlarging abdominal girth exerts upward pressure on the stomach, forcing the esophageal sphincter to open when the pressure exceeds its ability to stay shut. Not all causes of GERD are explained by these mechanisms but clearly the majority of cases are. GERD is therefore largely a disease of an unbalanced lifestyle and should usually be easily correctable. Instead, we ignore the root cause and look to pharmaceuticals to *manage* the problem.

Two of the most overused medications in this century are the proton pump inhibitors (PPIs) and histamine (H_2) blockers. These drugs do not address the underlying cause of GERD; they only manage the symptoms! Taking them neutralizes the acidic pH of the stomach but this violates intended physiology which requires that stomach acid maintain a pH of 2.5 for two critical reasons: 1) to hydrolyze and digest protein chains and 2) to destroy most bacteria inadvertently swallowed after entry into the body via the mouth or sinuses.

By using these medications heartburn symptoms may be relieved — not because the acid reflux has been corrected but because the pH of the stomach content has now been neutralized. This loss of the strong acidic environment within the stomach interferes with optimal protein digestion and can lead to the failure to kill some potentially harmful bacteria that enters the stomach.

Studies suggest that chronic use of proton pump inhibitors increase the risk of *Clostridium difficile* colitis, fractures likely due to calcium malabsorption, and both community-acquired and hospital-acquired pneumonias.[10] Furthermore, between 1975 and 2005, the incidence of GERD and esophageal adenocarcinoma increased fivefold in most Western countries.[11]

Chronic Acid States
- Acid Reflux
- Cancer
- Gout
- Kidney Stones
- Osteoporosis
- Dental Disease

We can do better. We can address the cause of this disease and eliminate the need for most people to depend on prescription medicine to manage disease symptoms that don't treat the underlying problem and can even mask cancer! The take-home message is: Restore equilibrium and physiology by lifestyle choices that return the body to a more balanced, alkaline state. Ionized water supports this effort.

Osteoporosis affects an estimated 75 million people in Europe, the U.S. and Japan[12]. One in three women over 50 will experience osteoporotic fractures at some point in their lifetime, as will one in five men[13,14,15].

Osteoporosis is associated with a high rate of spontaneous vertebral fractures resulting in debilitating pain, and hip fractures that carry a high risk of mortality within six months due to complications of immobility, infection and blood clots. By the early twenties human bones have reached their maximum density. From this point forward the activity of bone cells that dissolve bone minerals (osteoclasts) exceeds the activity of those that build it (osteoblasts), resulting in a slow, gradual loss of bone density.

The bones store 99 percent of the body's calcium in the form of calcium salts. Smoking, acidic states and inactivity accelerate the loss of these salts, thus weakening the bone matrix and leading first to osteopenia and later osteoporosis. Diets high in acidic stressors (i.e. soft drinks, high fructose corn syrup and other processed foods) as well as lifestyles that lack sufficient weight-bearing activity predispose the human body to this diseased state. A diet rich in alkaline foods (vegetables, beans, legumes and some fruits) and ionized water may be one of the simplest and safest ways to minimize this acidic stress. Alkaline, ionized water is a natural fit.

Cancer is another disease that seems to thrive in chronic acidic states. Dr. Otto Warburg's research in this area earned him a Nobel Prize in physiology in 1931. His conclusion was that cancer cannot grow in an oxygen-rich, alkaline environment. It is clear that cancer rates have risen dramatically in the last 50 years. Some argue that a longer life expectancy naturally raises the risk of developing cancer and explains why it appears there is more cancer — perhaps this is true. But this does not explain why Japanese natives, eating a diet high in vegetables, rice and fish have very low cancer rates, then quickly becomes susceptible to the Western cancers (i.e. colon, prostate, breast) within a few decades of adopting the American diet. Furthermore, this is not an observation unique to the Japanese. Many other non-industrialized countries can boast of low rates of cancer as well.[16]

Diets high in *animal protein* place an acidic burden on the body. Proteins are made up of acids, called amino acids. They are essential for our health because they are the building blocks of protein. We must include 10 of these amino acids in our diet because they are essential, we cannot synthesize them. Interestingly, from these 10 amino acids our biochemistry can synthesize the other 10 we need.

This almost seems to be a clue that we don't need too much of these acids, if half of what our body uses is made from the other 10 we require from our diet. For most individuals the recommended daily protein intake is generously estimated at 0.8 g/kg of ideal body weight. This can be achieved with very little animal protein in the daily diet. For an adult with an ideal body weight of 175 pounds, the daily protein need is only 63 grams, but could be as high as 120 grams if the individual exercises heavily or is trying to build additional muscle. This is not a high protein requirement.

We have simply been misinformed about these requirements and in the meantime have developed a love affair with meats and dairy products.

Gout is a common, painful joint inflammation that results from an accumulation of uric acid in affected joints. Gout is really a buildup of needle-sharp crystals created by either an overproduction or under-excretion of uric acid. Diets high in amino *acids* and nucleic *acids* (organ meats, etc.) and alcohol often predispose to this condition. Limiting the acidic dietary load and flushing the body and the kidneys with alkaline rich, ionized water would seem to be a simple solution to this issue. Because gout is also an inflammatory process, oxidative stress is involved in the disease process as well, further underscoring the potential benefit of hydrating tissues with free-radical quenching, antioxidant-rich water.

For unknown reasons, the number of people in the United States with *kidney stones* has been increasing over the past 30 years. In the late 1970s, less than four percent of the population suffered from kidney stones. By the early 1990s, the portion of the population with this disease had increased to more than five percent.

Kidney stones result from the accumulation of acids, especially amino acids, from diets high in protein. As the body attempts to buffer these acid loads, calcium is leached from bones — contributing to kidney stone formation. While the formation of kidney stones is not always this simple, mainstay treatments include limiting animal protein intake and drinking up to two quarts of water each day. Drinking alkaline water, which penetrates cells and tissues more effectively due to micro-clustering

36

features (see "Micro-clustering" section), is a logical, simple and potentially quite effective treatment.

Periodontal disease is characterized by the progressive loss of tissue surrounding and supporting the teeth. The process is initiated by the overgrowth of acid-producing bacteria that feed on sugars that bathe or stick to the teeth and gums. Although the pH of saliva is 6.0-7.4, this slightly acidic state aids in the breakdown of carbohydrates, which begins in the mouth. But when normal chemistry is violated long enough and acid loads extend beyond designed biochemistry, the acidic stress results in destruction of the periodontal structures.

One of the simplest treatments to support healthy teeth is a diet rich in raw foods and alkaline water. Those most predisposed to periodontal disease and cavities have repeated exposures of acidic states in their saliva from direct exposure to acids, especially those found in soft drinks (i.e. phosphoric acid) and indirectly from the acids produced by bacteria that feed on sugars that bathe the teeth (i.e. sticky candies and other sweets). Furthermore, saliva is continuously secreted from the salivary glands in the mouth to wash stronger acids away. With age, the salivary glands produce less saliva or can become dysfunctional, further putting the mouth in a more acidic state that can erode enamel and the periodontal tissues. Regular consumption of alkaline water is a simple way to keep the gums and teeth healthy and limit the buildup of plaque.

Hydration Stress

We are 70-75 percent water, one big biochemical reaction. The aging process seems to be associated with a relative loss of hydration. The elderly are believed to be only 65% water, while infants are very hydrated (75-80%). Due to the polar nature of water, it is the ideal solvent. We can survive for weeks without food but only days without water. We are much more likely to be dehydrated than hungry.

Dehydration States
Aging
Sleep
Constipation
Kidney stones
Some headaches

Dehydration Practices
Diuretics
Caffeine
Limited water intake
Dry Heat
Exercise

Yet, because we are not aware of the signals our body gives us, we often peer into the refrigerator, looking to quench our "hunger" with a food that is very hydrated, such as an orange, a melon, juice, a tomato, etc.

What we should do is drink 12-20 ounces of water first and then decide if we still feel hungry. Also, every morning we awaken in a slightly dehydrated state. Therefore, a simple and useful dietary practice is to drink water before eating breakfast, or any meal for that matter.

When we ignore the dehydration signals or fail to recognize dehydrating practices, we disrupt a delicate, but crucial balance. This is hydration stress.

Unfortunately, most of us ignore the subtle feedback our bodies give us. We begin each day dehydrated from the overnight loss of fluid through both urination and respiration. We don't even become aware of the thirst signal until we are five percent dehydrated. In addition to that, many of us take diuretics or drink caffeine, both of which dehydrate our tissues. For youngsters, dehydration states come about quicker due to the large surface area to total body mass ratio and the immature signaling of their thirst mechanism. If you watch young children on a soccer field or baseball diamond in the summertime, you will notice symptoms of dehydration and heat exhaustion --- fatigue, headache, nausea, vomiting, etc. If this state continues, they may quickly develop life-threatening heat stroke, characterized as a "broken cooling mechanism". Heat stroke presents with loss of sweating, elevated temperature, confusion and extreme irritability.

Bottom line, by hydrating with alkaline, antioxidant-rich and superior tissue- and cellular-penetrating water, we can bathe every cell, every tissue with the most predominant, important and healing molecule the body can use. Nothing could be simpler or more important than this single practice!

History of Ionized water

One of the earliest observations about the unique healing properties of water was first witnessed by residents in small villages around the world whose primary water source came from snow-capped, mountain runoff streams. The Alps, the Himalayan and Caucasus mountains have historically given rise to regions where area natives, who drank water from these streams, seemed to have fewer diseases and lived longer.

The Russians first observed and investigated the properties of this water, wondering if there was something unique in the water that might explain the apparent longevity and healing properties to residents who drank this water. They noted the water was alkaline (pH 8.5-9.5), high in oxidation-reduction potential (negative ORP), and micro-clustered in structure. Upon this discovery attempts were made to recreate this same water in the laboratory. Due to their awkwardly large size and cost they gave up on efforts to manufacture the machines to recreate this water for consumer use. However, in the early 1950s Japanese scientists picked up where the Russians left off. Within a few years the Japanese had manufactured a smaller, more portable and higher quality machine. It's been estimated that approximately 20 percent of Japanese households currently use water ionizers. They are also used in hospitals in Japan for treatment of cancer, heart disease, diabetes, gangrene and eczema.

The Chemistry of Water

Water is comprised of two hydrogen atoms and one oxygen atom. Hydrogen is the most abundant element in the universe and oxygen is the third most abundant (helium is the second). In the human body, elemental oxygen makes up 65 percent of total body weight, carbon 18 percent and hydrogen 10 percent. In other words, these three atoms (oxygen, hydrogen and carbon) make up 93 percent of the total weight of the body. It should be no surprise then that water, comprised of oxygen and hydrogen, is the most abundant and important molecule in the most complex of all life forms — the human body.

While we all recognize that H_2O is water, we should not assume that it is a simple molecule. We accept that temperature and pressure dictate whether water exists as a gas, liquid or a solid. Pollack and his team at the University of Washington have shown that cellular water can exist in a fourth state, a *liquid crystal*. Their research documents that water can layer along cellular surfaces creating an electric potential, charge differences, restricted vibrational frequencies and other features that impact cellular chemistry[17]. The liquid crystal property found also on surface water explains the strength of surface tension and why a small coin or an insect fail to sink on the surface of water.

Because of the chemistry of hydrogen and oxygen, water may be the most versatile chemical structure in the universe. It is without question the most vital since without it life could not exist. In fact, it is well accepted that living organisms originated in water. But what makes it so crucial to life?

The oxygen atom forms the center of water. At the center of the oxygen atom, within the nucleus, are eight neutrons ("n") and eight positively charged protons ("p").

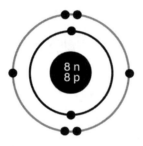

Surrounding this center is a cloud of negatively charged electrons pulled toward the nucleus by the positive charge of eight protons. As the diagram depicts, the inner shell surrounding the nucleus can hold two electrons and is always filled first by their strong attraction to the positively charged protons. The second (outer) shell contains six (three sets of two pairs) additional electrons, but is capable of holding a maximum of eight. This feature means that the oxygen atom is always seeking to fill this shell with two more electrons. To do this oxygen must steal two additional electrons from other atoms. Atoms like oxygen that do this are called *oxidizing agents* or *oxidants* because they steal electrons to satisfy the need to fill their shell.

By contrast, the hydrogen atom has only one proton (and one neutron) in its nucleus. This single proton exerts a relatively weak pull on the lone electron found in elemental hydrogen. Consequently, hydrogen's electron can easily be stolen or donated by the stronger pull from the eight protons in the nucleus of oxygen. Therefore, hydrogen donates its lone electron to other atoms with a stronger proton pull. For this purpose, hydrogen is referred to as a reducing agent or an "anti" oxidant. This unique chemistry renders oxygen an oxidant (a stealer of electrons) by nature, and hydrogen, a reductant (a donor of electrons). This fact further underscores the important atomic charge balance or oxidation-reduction potential that exists throughout all of nature and especially in nature's most crucial, life-sustaining molecule — water.

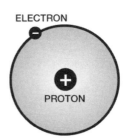

This attraction for electrons renders oxygen relatively negatively charged on one end and relatively positively charged on the other due to the location of the hydrogen atoms that bind to it. This results in the polarity of water, which allows the water molecule to act like a magnet, which can then attract other minerals and chemicals. For this reason, water is the ideal solvent, attracting itself to other positively or negatively charged molecules AND to other water molecules.

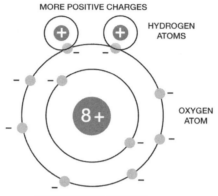

MORE POSITIVE CHARGES

HYDROGEN ATOMS

8 +

OXYGEN ATOM

MORE NEGATIVE CHARGES

Another key feature of water is that H_2O does not exist ONLY as this molecule. It is important to note that some oxygen atoms are "dissolved" in water and are referred to as Dissolved Oxygen (DO) or "Active Oxygen". This is simply oxygen (O_2) gas. Likewise, water also contains a certain amount of free Dissolved Hydrogen (DH) atoms, also known as "Active Hydrogen" or Hydrogen (H_2) gas. These are fundamental conditions of water.

In commercial water ionizers freshly made alkaline water will contain H_2 gas, charged with two electrons per H_2 molecule. Some H_2 gas will quickly dissipate into the atmosphere, while much of it will remain in solution, especially if the water is kept cool and in a closed container. Heating alkaline water and the passage of time both result in a loss of electron-rich, Active Hydrogen to the atmosphere. For this reason, alkaline water, loaded with anti-oxidant properties is best when freshly made and used.

On the other hand, acid water contains O_2 gas, some of which will quickly dissipate into the atmosphere. What remains in the acid solution, will serve as an oxidant capable of destroying many common pathogens. It is best when applied topically and should not be used internally. The same storage recommendations apply for acid water, although it is also most effective when used from a freshly made source.

What this means is that water contains some dissolved oxygen atoms and some dissolved hydrogen atoms. Furthermore, *when water holds more dissolved hydrogen atoms, (depicted as H, not H+, which is acidic) it is enriched in free electrons, making it a powerful antioxidant.* This is the feature noted in the water from many of the world's highest mountain streams.

For electrons to be shifted from one molecule to another minerals are needed. It has been reported that some minerals support the structure of water and others favor the loss of that structure. Remember, energy, chemistry and life is all about balance!

The following table illustrates this balance. In biological systems Sodium and Chloride as well as Calcium and Magnesium, are often balanced to establish both electro-chemical and structural

45

equilibrium. It is noteworthy to point out that while magnesium and potassium are crucial cellular minerals, aluminum, chloride, and fluoride are minerals that have recently come under criticism for health-compromising features. Yet, we continue to find high levels of chloride and fluoride in municipal water supplies.

Structure-making ions			Structure-breaking ions		
Name	**Ion**	**Eww***	**Name**	**Ion**	**Eww**
Calcium	Ca^{2+}	32.2	Magnesium	Mg^{2+}	-8.8
Lithium	Li^{2+}	27.2	Potassium	K^+	-3.8
Sodium	Na^+	3.3	Aluminum	Al^{3+}	-313.4
Zinc	Zn^{2+}	50.6	Chloride	Cl^-	-7.5
Iron	Fe^{3+}	51.9	Fluoride	Fl^-	-18.8
Molecular movement is made difficult due to the water molecule's decreased degree of freedom			Molecular movement is facilitated due to the water molecule's increased degree of freedom		

*Eww is the interaction energy (kJ/mol) between water molecules in solution.[18]

The chemistry is simple. If enough energy can be supplied to mineral-rich water by either the process of electrolysis, or the friction of cold water crashing over mineral rocks as it flows at high speeds down mountains, many of the water molecules can be split by this reaction:

$$H_2O \rightarrow HO \cdot + H^+ + e^-$$

Active oxygen species such as $^1O_2$, O_2^-, H_2O_2 or HO $\cdot$ are free radicals and can result in sickness if not scavenged by antioxidants or active hydrogen, H_2 ($2H^+ + 2e^-$), as shown below:

$$O_2 + e^- \rightarrow O_2^-$$
$$O_2^- + 2H^+ + e^- \rightarrow H_2O_2$$
$$H_2O_2 + e^- \rightarrow HO \cdot + HO^-$$
$$HO \cdot + H^+ + e^- \rightarrow H_2O$$
$$HO^- + H^+ \rightarrow H_2O$$

Consequently, ionized reduced water obtained from electrolysis contains many unique features when compared to everyday tap water, which, as shown below by a positive ORP, is very oxidizing.[18]

	DO (ppm)	DH (ppb)	ORP (mV)	pH
Tap water	10.0	2.3 − 2.6	**+652**	7.5
Reduced Water	8.6	690 -720	-247	10.3

Electrolysis

The chemsitry of electrolysis was discovered by Michael Faraday (1791-1867). In the process, electrons are added (reduction) at the cathode side of a semi-permeable membrane and electrons are removed (oxidation) at the anode.

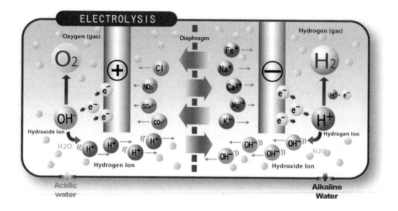

ANODE reaction

$$2H_2O ==> O_2(g) + 4H^+ + 4e^-$$

CATHODE reaction

$$4H_2O + 4e^- ==> 2H_2(g) + 4OH^-$$

Electrolysis takes place via a "restructuring" of water through a process of ionization. In most

48

commercial ionizers, water is first run through a high-grade filter to remove trace organic and inorganic contaminants and microbes that sometimes make their way into municipal water supplies. This filtered water is then passed over a series of platinum-coated titanium plates (platinum acts as a catalyst) in the presence of trace amounts of the commonly present ions such as calcium, magnesium, and sodium that provide a chemical charge through which the electrical current can be transmitted. In the absence of these minerals, as in the case of reverse osmosis water, the electrolysis process cannot proceed, hence the term "dead water." With the electrical potential from these ions, the plates are charged with approximately 220 watts of electrical energy from an external source. The process of electrolysis uses high amounts of energy in the presence of the catalyst (the platinum-coated plates) to change the chemical structure of water in three ways:

1. pH — Splitting of water into hydrogen (H^+) ions and hydroxyl (OH^-) ions

2. ORP — Generation of free electrons from platinum nanoparticles associating with hydrogen ion to form "Active Hydrogen"

3. Micro-clustering — Reduction in the nuclear magnetic resonance energy of the H_2O molecule

As previously mentioned the cathode reaction generates Active Hydrogen (H_2 gas) and hydroxyl ions, resulting in an electron-donating, alkaline solution. On the other hand, the anode reaction generates Active Oxygen (O_2 gas) and hydrogen ions resulting in an oxidizing, acidic solution. In other words, after the source water undergoes electrolysis, two separate types of waters emerge from separate hoses in all ionizing units. **Since the pH range covers a scale from 0-14, the combined pH of both water types generated must equal 14. For example, if one hose generates water with an alkaline pH of 8.5, the other hose will deliver water with a pH of 5.5.**

Alkaline water, rich in antioxidants (from Active Hydrogen) is intended for internal use to support cellular healing by alkalizing, hydrating and neutralizing free radical damage. Acid water, rich in oxidizing agents (from Active Oxygen) is ideal for topical use only because these features are highly bactericidal due to both their low pH and oxidizing effect on infectious microbes

pH (Potential Hydrogen)

In the chemistry of electrolysis, by convention, the positively charged hydrogen (H^+) ions flow towards the anode while the negatively charged hydroxyl (OH^-) ions flow towards the cathode. Consequently, electrolysis separates these components of H_2O. The hydrogen (H^+) ions constitute the "acid" component of the water and the hydroxyl (OH^-) ions make up the "alkaline" component.

pH   7.0 is neutral, equal (H^+) & (OH^-) ions
pH   2.5 is very acidic, many (H^+) ions
pH 11.5 is very basic, many (OH^-) ions

The term pH stands for "potential Hydrogen." The more hydrogen (H^+) ions are concentrated in a solution, the more acidic it is. While the full pH scale range is from 0 to 14, anything below a pH of seven is considered acidic and anything above seven is considered alkaline (or basic).

Therefore a solution with a pH of 2.5 is much more acidic and has much more hydrogen (H^+) ions than a solution of 6.5. Likewise, a pH of 11.5 has many more hydroxyl (OH^-) ions and is therefore much more alkaline than a pH of 7.5.

There is a logarithmic relationship with reference to pH scale. For example, for every one point difference in pH there is a 10-fold difference in the number of ions present. Put another way:

pH 6 has 10 times more hydrogen (H^+) ions than a pH of 7
pH 5 has 100 times more hydrogen (H^+) ions than a pH of 7
pH 4 has 1,000 times more hydrogen (H^+) ions than a pH of 7
pH 3 has 10,000 times more hydrogen (H^+) ions than a pH of 7
pH 2 has 100,000 times more hydrogen (H^+) ions than a pH of 7
pH 1 has 1,000,000 times more hydrogen (H^+) ions than a pH of 7

likewise;

pH 8 has 10 times more hydroxyl (OH^-) ions than a pH of 7
pH 9 has 100 times more hydroxyl (OH^-) ions than a pH of 7
pH 10 has 1,000 times more hydroxyl (OH^-) ions than a pH of 7
pH 11 has 10,000 times more hydroxyl (OH^-) ions than a pH of 7
pH 12 has 100,000 times more hydroxyl (OH^-) ions than a pH of 7
pH 13 has 1,000,000 times more hydroxyl (OH^-) ions than a pH of 7

Therefore, by nature both acid and alkaline water can be created as electrolysis moves electrons and separates acid from alkaline on each side of the membrane. Since the total pH must total 14, whatever alkaline pH number is selected to run out of the alkaline hose, the water coming from the acidic hose, by convention, must have a pH, that when combined with the alkaline pH, equals 14.

Oxidation-Reduction Potential (ORP)

Most hydrogen in nature is found as hydrogen gas (H_2) or as hydrogen ion (H^+), where the electron is absent because the single proton in the nucleus of hydrogen exerts a weak pull to hold onto the electron. Active Hydrogen is a hydrogen atom that holds its electron. This extra electron is derived from nanoparticles created through the electrolysis process during which platinum-coated plates are charged with an electrical current.[19]

Water that is rich in active hydrogen will therefore have a negative ORP. The more negative the ORP value, the more free-radical neutralizing electrons the water contains and the stronger its antioxidant properties. This extra electron is able to react with other compounds in the body to control Redox reactions. In essence, these electrons create an electric field inside the cell and serve as a rich source of antioxidants that can neutralize some of the harmful effects of free radicals, helping to restore the health and balance of the cell.

By contrast, most bottled waters, sports drinks and certainly soft drinks have highly positive ORP values. These drinks are oxidizing, pulling electrons, *creating* free radicals and contributing to oxidative stress. Their consumption should be minimized in your quest towards optimal health.

Micro-clustering

Perhaps one of the most significant features of ionized water is its ability to hydrate cells. The precise explanation for this mechanism has not been clearly established. Since we now understand that water penetrates cell membranes through specific protein channels, it is conceivable that in a state of oxidative stress these protein pores may become damaged and somewhat dysfunctional. This could theoretically impair cellular hydration. By drinking anti-oxidant rich alkaline water it is not a stretch to imagine that these oxidized protein channels could be restored to their healthy state, allowing for improved entry of water into the cell, thus allowing optimal cellular hydration.

Another theory proposed by two different groups maintains that the electrolysis process lowers the vibratory frequency of the water molecule.[20,21] This permits a closer association between molecules primarily forming a complex of six water molecules bound by the polar nature of these molecules. This is referred to as *hexagonal water* or a *micro-cluster.*

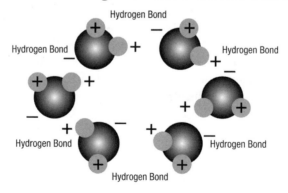

To understand this concept requires a recognition that every element, every atom, has a vibrational frequency. In other words, every atom vibrates or resonates. This resonating quality is measured by Nuclear Magnetic Resonance (NMR). For example, if our ears were capable of detecting this frequency, we could "hear" the unique sound of each atom. If our sensory system was keen enough, we could also feel the vibrations of each atom. Since all matter is made up of various atoms, each atom has its own unique vibration frequency.

When atoms mix with other atoms to form molecules, they take on a new vibrational energy or resonance. Just like the keys of a piano, one key produces one sound, but multiple keys struck simultaneously produce a nearly infinite number of frequencies, some chords with frequencies (vibrational energies) that match or resonant, or some that don't match, creating dissonant energies.

During the electrolysis process electrical charges change the vibrational frequency (Nuclear Magnetic Resonance or NMR) of the H_2O molecule. In essence, as a result of the energy input by electrolysis, water molecules vibrate at a much lower frequency, allowing them to cluster together more tightly and in a smaller cluster (a micro-cluster) of typically five or six H_2O molecules, compared to the more typical cluster size of 10 to 13 molecules. Smaller water molecule clusters are proposed to allow for simpler and faster penetration both in and out of cell membranes, not only enhancing cellular hydration, but also aiding in the removal of cellular waste. This feature of resonating, vibrating energy is measured in Hertz (Hz) as shown below.[22] The lower the NMR reading, the smaller the clusters as shown below:

Bottled mineral water	= 90-100 Hz
Normal tap water	~ 128 Hz
Reverse osmosis	~ 128 Hz
Distilled water	~ 128 Hz
Ionized water	= 42.3 Hz

Whatever the mechanism, ionized water clearly appears to hydrate tissues extremely well. The fact that the precise mechanism has not been widely accepted by the scientific community, does not disprove the observation of improved cellular hydration. At the very least, the critical thinker would be wise to research and follow future literature in this arena with an open mind.

Frequently Asked Questions

Won't my stomach just neutralize alkaline water once it reaches the acidic stomach?

This appears to be a logical conclusion, but normal physiology suggests that the stomach is not always acidic. Hydrochloric acid is released from parietal cells lining the stomach in response to the presence of both protein and mechanical stretching of the stomach. Water, like alcohol, is absorbed directly across the lining of the stomach without stimulating the release of hydrochloric acid. This suggests that if a person drinks alkaline water before meals when the stomach is empty it will be quickly absorbed and circulated throughout the body.

Can I just use baking soda to alkalize my water?

Baking soda is sodium bicarbonate. Bicarbonate is one of the body's major fluid buffers. This seems to be a logical question — in fact, bicarbonate was recently added to one of the newest acid reflux medications as an adjunct to treat acid reflux and neutralize the acidic stomach pH. Electrolyzed, ionized water provides much more than an alkaline hydrating source. It is rich in antioxidant potential and it is micro-clustered, allowing the water to penetrate cells much more effectively, introducing both anti-oxidant and alkaline characteristics to cells desperately in need of relief from oxidative and acidic stress.

The body has multiple buffer systems, why should I expect alkaline water to make a difference?

This is an excellent question that demonstrates sound logic and recognition of the body's major buffering systems. The answer lies in supporting the body's inherent, built-in buffering systems. Remember, the lungs quickly buffer the pH of blood by changing the respiratory rate. The kidneys buffer the blood by excreting hydrogen ions in the urine and absorbing bicarbonate back into the blood. Fluid buffers like bicarbonate and proteins operate much more slowly. Neither the kidneys nor the fluid buffers were designed with the capacity to handle long-term management of the strongly acidic states our bodies are in as a result of poor eating habits, toxic environmental exposure, and extreme stress many of us endure in our daily lives. An alkaline water source closely resembling the pH of some of nature's best foods can help offset many of these challenges.

Should I drink water with a pH of 2.5 to aid stomach digestion, particularly of protein?

No. When drinking water produced by an ionizer, the process of electrolysis, by its very chemistry, adds electrons to the alkaline water and strips them from the acidic water. Therefore, the acidic water created from electrolysis is oxidizing. When it is measured with an Oxidation Reduction Potential meter, it will measure very positive (oxidizing). This is the very property that renders acidic water bactericidal (bacteria killing), an oxidizing state. Oxidizing products, even water, do not belong in the body as they can directly damage healthy tissue. No one would ever recommend drinking hydrogen peroxide — it has a similar oxidation effect and can injure healthy tissue. Some medical professionals even warn against frequent application of hydrogen peroxide on the skin because it not only destroys bacteria but also healthy tissue if used in excess.

To aid digestion there are some easy things to do: slow down when you're eating and chew each bite of food well before swallowing it. Chewing stimulates saliva release and applies mechanical pressure to break the food apart to initiate digestion. Food should be swallowed after it becomes a pasty consistency. For example, if you eat peanuts, chew them to the consistency of peanut butter before swallowing. Eat more of a plant-based diet and try to avoid low-fiber, processed foods that tend to be high in fats, corn syrups and other artificial agents. Keep your meals smaller.

Sorry mom… but try to forget what you might have been told when growing up about finishing everything on your plate. As a society we tend to overeat and current statistics show that more than 60% of the U.S. population is overweight.

Should I drink 11.5 pH water to neutralize my acid reflux?

No, pH 9.5 water would be better. While this approach has the potential to help relieve symptoms, it does not address the underlying problem with physiology. My suggestion is to follow the ideas presented in the section under acid reflux. ALWAYS try to address the root cause of disease and dysfunction. Shortcutting our own physiology is a prescription for disaster!

Can infants drink alkaline water?

The real question is what should infants drink and why? Physiology and nature have answered this question. Infants should ideally nurse from their mothers. The process of milk production in mothers, where nutrients are shuttled from the mother to her breast milk to provide the highest quality nutrients for her young, creates the perfect food for infants.

In some cases mothers are not able to nurse, necessitating the practice of supplementing with formula. Since the pH of mother's milk ranges from 7.2-7.4, it is logical to conclude that ionized water in this pH range is ideal for reconstituting formula because it is free of the contaminates and chlorine found in tap water.

Why do I need to drink pH 7.0 water when I take prescription medications?

Ionized water that is pH 7.0 does not support the chemistry that enhances cellular hydration. Medications were designed to be bioavailable to tissues based upon calculations of dissociation constants that are based, not upon ionized water with a low NMR or highly negative ORP, but on tap water with a higher NMR and more neutral ORP. Drink only pH 7.0 water with medications and through the next hour to ensure that predicted steady state levels are maintained as indicated by the manufacturer.

Can I take nutritional supplements with ionized water?

Absolutely. In fact, it is believed that the superior hydrating features of the water will deliver the nutrients of the supplement into the cell at a much higher rate and with better efficiency than with tap water. You may be able to reduce the amount of supplements you take.

Is there any danger in drinking too much water?

Yes. There is a condition called Hyponatremia — commonly referred to as "Water Intoxication" that results from excessive water consumption. When water intake is excessive, and this can be highly dependent upon individual circumstances, blood sodium levels can become diluted. If sodium levels drop too low the individual can become extremely weak, tired, suffer muscle cramps, seizures or brain swelling. A 2005 study in the *New England Journal of Medicine* found that close to one sixth of marathon runners develop some degree of *Hyponatremia*. This is a rare medical condition but it can happen with overconsumption or water or with extreme dehydration. The analogy of changing the water of a fish tank is useful here; if you change too much water in a fish tank at one time, it can shock the fish and kill them. Change your water slowly and consistently. To be safe, do not exceed more than two to three gallons per day of ionized water. The rule of thumb is to drink one-half ounce of water per pound of body weight per day.

Are there any medical conditions that require cautious use of alkaline water?

Yes. Individuals with kidney failure should proceed with caution and consult their physician; however this group is unquestionably highly acidic and needs the benefits of alkalization, cellular hydration and antioxidant support. Nevertheless, hydrate slowly and with patience.

Individuals with psychosis, who are taking anti-psychotic medications, should always be closely monitored by a physician. They are at the biggest risk of water intoxication. Ionized water is the ideal hydrating source for this group. However their intake should be monitored closely and they should seek medical supervision to assure they do not develop Hyponatremia.

Individuals with Congestive Heart Failure are often on restricted fluid intake and reduced sodium load. If they are closely monitoring their sodium levels, there should be no reason alkaline water cannot be the source of water for this group. However, they should consult their physician before implementing the ionized water into their diet.

How can I get my medical doctor to listen to me when I talk about ionized water?

First, respect your doctor's time. Second, if you are granted time, present a well-rehearsed 60 second demonstration illustrating either the ORP, or hydrating properties of the water. Third, and most importantly, doctors want to see scientific evidence to be reassured that what they are being told is not just your personal testimonial, especially if you're not a peer with a medical degree. That's one of the reasons I wrote this book. I wanted to help my peers and streamline their exposure process by sharing what I've learned. Don't get caught up in the hype of your testimonial stories; it will turn off the critical thinker who is looking for evidence. Keep the testimonials brief and emphasize the science that supports your testimony.

How could ionized water help my athletic performance?

Exercise results in the buildup of metabolic acids. Much of these acids are removed by respiration but muscles in particular build up lactic acid that contributes to fatigue and impairs performance. By drinking water which contains Active Hydrogen, cellular oxidative stress can quickly be reduced, acidic byproducts like lactic acid can be neutralized and stressed cells can quickly become rehydrated. Water is a necessary component of cellular respiration and nowhere is drinking it more important than in exercising fatigued muscles. *The coach who instructs his team to drink only ionized water is a wise coach and will see better recovery of the athlete both during practice and competition.* I believe ionized water is the best sports nutrition supplement of this century!

Are there any simple ways to explain how ionized water might improve chronic diseases?

- Oxidative structural damage to collagen cross-links _ less skin elasticity_ wrinkles
- Oxidative structural damage to elastin protein _ stiffer arterial walls _ hypertension
- Oxidative structural damage to arterial wall lining _ atherosclerosis
- Oxidative damage to DNA/RNA _ mutations, inefficient repair processes and cancer
- Oxidative structural damage to Insulin Receptor _ diabetes

What should I look for in a water ionizer?

When selecting an ionizer it may be helpful to keep the following in mind:

1. A high quality product will probably not be the least expensive. Be willing to invest in your health.

2. Select a vendor with an established track record. Be cautious of the new kid on the block.

3. Look for industry awards and certifications to ensure quality.

4. A large portion of the cost and quality of an ionizer is found in its interior. Machines with high quality "guts," i.e., platinum-coated titanium plates with a large surface area, will cost more up front but will consistently produce the healthiest water and last the longest.

5. Most of the less expensive units produce a very slow stream of water.

6. Many of the warranties on inexpensive units are void if the machine is used in areas with hard water (80% of the U.S. has hard water).

7. Many of the warranties on inexpensive units are void if the machine is used commercially.

8. All units will make both alkaline and acidic water. But look for an ionizer that can create strong acidic water with a pH of 2.6 or lower so the bactericidal features will exist.

9. Do your homework on the details such as warranty, return policies and customer support.

10. Be cautious of some of the critiques found on the Internet. They typically lack any credible scientific basis and are written by a biased party with something to gain.

11. Become educated before making your purchase. Attend demonstrations and learn as much as you can first. Talk with others who actually own the model you're thinking of purchasing and get their feedback.

12. Understand that most units will be sold through direct sales marketing. It's not a product you'll find on the shelf of your local big box retailer.

13. Be wary of any vendor that obligates you to sell anything to purchase your unit. Becoming a company distributor should be optional.

14. Ionizers require mineral rich water to generate the many beneficial features we've discussed. If your source water is mineral-free, like reverse osmosis water, your unit will not work properly unless you add back a sufficient amount of minerals to the water.

15. Depending on your source water, you may want to purchase pre-filters to extend the life of the filter in the ionizer and deal with other potential contamination issues like fluoride or other contaminants that can exist in well water.

16. Generally speaking, hard water provides better ions for the best ORP values. It is preferred over a soft water supply. But if your water is too hard, it can cause problems for the ionizer by coating the plates with calcium deposits (like you see in your shower and sink).

17. ORP values decline quickly. When possible, it is best to fill a glass of ionized water and drink it immediately. While I have found a container that does help retain ORP values for a couple of days, when stored in plastic bottles the ORP value will typically drop by 50 percent within 24 hours, and revert back to its original state within 48 hours. Micro-clustering features and pH values decline more slowly, depending on the water's exposure to heat and light. By investing in a high-quality machine you will create higher ORP water to begin with, thus it will retain its ORP values longer. This is very important if you're sharing water with friends and family.

18. With a good ORP meter and pH meter, you can do your own testing to determine how long the various qualities of the water last with your source water and machine.

Final Thoughts
Keys to Healing

To enjoy good health we must understand and comply with the lesson nature teaches us —BALANCE! It is clear that the balance between oxidation and reduction is the core of both health and disease. Many lifestyle choices are inherently stressful, while others are additional burdens to which we consciously or even unconsciously submit ourselves. But consequences are consequences. The laws of nature will not, they cannot, be violated.

Ionized water plays a significant role in restoring the oxidation-reduction balance. But let us also assume greater personal responsibility for the foods we eat, the toxic exposures to which we submit ourselves, and even the negative, self-defeating thoughts, emotions and behaviors we often fall victim to. They all affect our health. They all impact our healing.

The famous physician Claude Bernard made this insightful statement: "The terrain is everything; the germ is nothing." On his death bed Louis Pasteur even recanted his Germ Theory: "It's the terrain, not the germ." When it comes to healing, the same principle applies; we must first clean up our cellular environment so healing can occur. Below is a list of simple, profoundly critical solutions to cleaning up our cellular environment to help support a healing biochemistry:

1. Minimize sources of oxidative stress from your diet and lifestyle

2. Balance oxidative stress with antioxidants

3. Increase consumption of nature's plant-based foods

4. Learn about and take high-quality supplements

5. Exercise every day

6. Reduce emotional stress

7. Laugh, love, play, serve others

8. HAVE AN OPEN MIND AND AN OPEN MOUTH — DRINK ALKALINE, IONIZED MICROCLUSTERED WATER DAILY!

Research & Additional Reading

Ther Apher Dial. 2009 Jun;13(3):220-4.

Ionized alkaline water: new strategy for management of metabolic acidosis in experimental animals.

Abol-Enein H, Gheith OA, Barakat N, Nour E, Sharaf AE.
Department of Urology, El Mansoura Urology and Nephrology Center, Mansoura University, 72 Gomhoria Street, Mansoura, Egypt.

Abstract
Metabolic acidosis can occur as a result of either the accumulation of endogenous acids or loss of bicarbonate from the gastrointestinal tract or the kidney, which represent common causes of metabolic acidosis. The appropriate treatment of acute metabolic acidosis has been very controversial. Ionized alkaline water was not evaluated in such groups of patients in spite of its safety and reported benefits. So, we aimed to assess its efficacy in the management of metabolic acidosis in animal models. Two models of metabolic acidosis were created in dogs and rats. The first model of renal failure was induced by ligation of both ureters; and the second model was induced by urinary diversion to gut (gastrointestinal bicarbonate loss model). Both models were subjected to ionized alkaline water (orally and by hemodialysis). Dogs with renal failure were assigned to two groups according to the type of dialysate utilized during hemodialysis sessions, the first was utilizing alkaline water and the second was utilizing conventional water. Another two groups of animals with urinary diversion were arranged to receive oral alkaline water and tap water. In renal failure animal models, acid-base parameters improved significantly after hemodialysis with ionized alkaline water compared with the conventional water treated with reverse osmosis (RO). Similar results were observed in urinary diversion models as there was significant improvement of both the partial pressure of carbon dioxide and serum bicarbonate (P = 0.007 and 0.001 respectively) after utilizing alkaline water orally. **Alkaline ionized water can be considered as a major safe strategy in the management of metabolic acidosis secondary to renal failure or dialysis or urinary diversion. Human studies are indicated in the near future to confirm this issue in humans.**

Biosci Biotechnol Biochem. 2006 Jan;70(1):31-7.

Anti-diabetic effect of alkaline-reduced water on OLETF rats.

Jin D, Ryu SH, Kim HW, Yang EJ, Lim SJ, Ryang YS, Chung CH, Park SK, Lee KJ. Department of Microbiology, Wonju College of Medicine, Yonsei University, Korea.

Abstract

Alkaline-reduced water (ARW) is known to exert several anti-cancer effects, as well as to scavenge reactive oxygen species (ROS) and reduce blood-glucose levels. This study was performed in order to determine the effects of ARW on the control of spontaneous diabetes in Otsuka Long-Evans Tokushima Fatty (OLETF) rats. We assigned 16 male OLETF rats (4 wk) to two groups: an experimental group, which was given ARW, and a control group, which received laboratory tap water. From week 6 to 32, the body weight, lipid composition, and glucose levels in the blood of the rats were measured. The glucose levels of both groups tended to increase. However, the ARW group's glucose levels were significantly lower than those of the control group after 12 weeks (p<0.05). **The total cholesterol and triglyceride levels in the ARW group were found to be significantly lower than those of the control group during the experimental period. These results suggest that ARW spurred the growth of OLETF rats during the growth stage, and that long-term ingestion of ARW resulted in a reduction in the levels of glucose, triglycerides, and total cholesterol in the blood.**

J Int Soc Life Inf Sci; Vol 22, No. 2, 302-305, 2004

Anticancer Effect of Alkaline Reduced Water

Kyu-Jae LEE[1,2], Seung-Kyu PARK[1,2], Jae-Won KIM[1], Gwang-Young KIM[1], Young-Suk RYANG[5], Geun-Ha KIM [1], Hyun-Cheol CHO[3], Soo-Kie KIM[2,3], and Hyun-Won KIM[2,4]

[1] Dept. of Parasitology, [2] Institute of Basic Medical Sciences, [3] Dept. of Microbiology, [4] Dept. of Biochemistry, Wonju College of Medicine, Yonsei Univ. (Wonju , Korea) [5]Dept. of Biomedical Laboratory Science and Institute of Health Science, College of Health Science, Yonsei Univ. (Wonju , Korea)

Abstract:
Certain minerals can produce alkaline reduced water with high pH and low oxidation-reduction potential (ORP) when dissolved in water. Alkaline reduced water (ARW) showed significant anticancer effect. When B16 melanoma cells were inoculated subcutaneously and intra-peritoneally, C56BL/6 mice fed with ARW showed tumor growth delay and the survival span was significantly lengthened. ARW also showed the inhibition of metastasis by reducing the numbers of B16 melanoma colonies when injected through tail vein. The amount of reactive oxygen species (ROS) was very reduced when fed with ARW except for spleen, which is a major organ for immunity. Even for normal mice, ARW intake invoked systemic cytokines, such as, Th1 (IFN-g, IL-12) and Th2 (IL-4, IL-5), suggesting strong immuno-modulation effect. Both ROS scavenging effect and immuno-modulation effect might be responsible for anticancer effect of alkaline reduced water.

Introduction
Reactive oxygen species (ROS) or free radicals are one of the major offenders to render oxidative damage to biological macromolecules. These unstable ROS are known to cause or aggravate a variety of incurable diseases such as cancer, cardiovascular diseases, neurodegenerative diseases as well as aging. The cellular radical-scavengers such as superoxide dismutase, catalase, glutathione peroxidase are natural defense system against ROS. External source of anti-oxidative protection include antioxidant vitamins C and E, carotene and carotenoids as well as minerals such as selenium and zinc. Great efforts have been made in an attempt to find safe and potent natural antioxidants.

Biological & Pharmaceutical Bulletin. 2008 Jan;31(1):19-26

Inhibitory effect of electrolyzed reduced water on tumor angiogenesis

Ye J, Li Y, Hamasaki T, Nakamichi N, Komatsu T, Kashiwagi T, Teruya K, Nishikawa R, Kawahara T, Osada K, Toh K, Abe M, Tian H, Kabayama S, Otsubo K, Morisawa S, Katakura Y, Shirahata S.
Graduate School of Systems Life Sciences, Kyushu University, Higashi-ku, Fukuoka 812-8581, Japan

Vascular endothelial growth factor (VEGF) is a key mediator of tumor angiogenesis. **Tumor cells are exposed to higher oxidative stress compared to normal cells. Numerous reports have demonstrated that the intracellular redox (oxidation/reduction, ORP) state is closely associated with the pattern of VEGF expression. Electrolyzed reduced water (ERW) produced near the cathode during the electrolysis of water scavenged intracellular H_2O_2 and decreased the release of H_2O_2 from a human lung adenocarcinoma cell line**, A549, and down-regulated both VEGF transcription and protein secretion in a time-dependent manner. To investigate the signal transduction pathway involved in regulating VEGF expression, mitogen-activated kinase (MAPK) specific inhibitors, SB203580 (APK inhibitor), PD98059 (ERK1/2 inhibitor) and JNKi (c-Jun N-terminal protein kinase inp38 Mhibitor) were applied. The results showed that only PD98059 blocks VEGF expression, suggesting an important role for ERK1/2 in regulating VEGF expression in A549 cells. As well, ERW inhibited the activation of extracellular signal-regulated kinase (ERK) in a time-dependent manner. Co-culture experiments to analyze in vitro tubule formation assay revealed that A549 cell-derived conditioned medium significantly stimulated the formation of vascular tubules in all analyzed parameters; tubule total area, tubule junction, number of tubules, and total tubule length. ERW counteracted the effect of A549 cell-conditioned medium and decreased total tube length (p<0.01). **The present study demonstrated that ERW down-regulated VEGF gene transcription and protein secretion through inactivation of ERK.**

Biochem Biophys Res Commun 1997 May 8;234(1):269-74.

Electrolyzed-reduced water scavenges active oxygen species and protects DNA from oxidative damage.

Shirahata S, Kabayama S, Nakano M, Miura T, Kusumoto K, Gotoh M, Hayashi H, Otsubo K, Morisawa S, Katakura Y.
Institute of Cellular Regulation Technology, Graduate School of Genetic Resources Technology, Kyushu University, Fukuoka, Japan.
sirahata@grt.kyushu-u.ac.jp

Active oxygen species or free radicals are considered to cause extensive oxidative damage to biological macromolecules, which brings about a variety of diseases as well as aging. The ideal scavenger for active oxygen should be 'active hydrogen'. 'Active hydrogen' can be produced in reduced water near the cathode during electrolysis of water. Reduced water exhibits high pH, low dissolved oxygen (DO), extremely high dissolved molecular hydrogen (DH), and extremely negative redox potential (RP) values. Strongly electrolyzed-reduced water, as well as ascorbic acid, (+)-catechin and tannic acid, completely scavenged $O._2^-$ produced by the hypoxanthine-xanthine oxidase (HX-XOD) system in sodium phosphate buffer (pH 7.0). The superoxide dismutase (SOD)-like activity of reduced water is stable at 4 degrees C for over a month and was not lost even after neutralization, repeated freezing and melting, deflation with sonication, vigorous mixing, boiling, repeated filtration, or closed autoclaving, but was lost by opened autoclaving or by closed autoclaving in the presence of tungsten trioxide which efficiently adsorbs active atomic hydrogen. Water bubbled with hydrogen gas exhibited low DO, extremely high DH and extremely low RP values, as does reduced water, but it has no SOD-like activity. These results suggest that the SOD-like activity of reduced water is not due to the dissolved molecular hydrogen but due to the dissolved atomic hydrogen (active hydrogen). Although SOD accumulated H2O2 when added to the HX-XOD system, reduced water decreased the amount of H2O2 produced by XOD. Reduced water, as well as catalase and ascorbic acid, could directly scavenge H2O2. **Reduced water suppresses single-strand breakage of DNA by active oxygen species produced by the Cu(II)-catalyzed oxidation of ascorbic acid in a dose-dependent manner, suggesting that reduced water can scavenge not only O_2^- and H_2O_2, but also $^1O_2$ and $\cdot OH$.**

Cytotechnology. 2005 Jan;47(1-3):97-105.

Electrolyzed Reduced Water Supplemented with Platinum Nanoparticles Suppresses Promotion of Two-stage Cell Transformation.

Nishikawa R, Teruya K, Katakura Y, Osada K, Hamasaki T, Kashiwagi T, Komatsu T, Li Y, Ye J, Ichikawa A, Otsubo K, Morisawa S, Xu Q, Shirahata S.
Department of Genetic Resources Technology, Faculty of Agriculture, Kyushu University, 6-10-1 Hakozaki, 812-8581, Higashi-ku, Fukuoka, Japan.

Abstract
In the two-stage cell transformation theory, cancer cells first receive initiation, which is mainly caused by DNA damage, and then promotion, which enhances transformation. Murine Balb/c 3T3 cells are widely used for transformation experiments because they lose contact inhibition ability when transformed. **Electrolyzed reduced water (ERW), which is produced near a cathode during electrolysis of water, is an alkaline drinking water that is beneficial to health. ERW contains a high concentration of dissolved hydrogen and scavenge reactive oxygen species (ROS), along with a small amount of platinum (Pt) nanoparticles (Pt nps) derived from Pt-coated titanium electrodes.** Pt nps stably disperse in aqueous solution for a long time, and convert hydrogen molecules to active hydrogen (atomic hydrogen) that can scavenge ROS. Therefore, ERW supplemented with synthesized Pt nps is a model strong reduced water. This is the first report that ERW supplemented with synthesized Pt nps strongly prevents transformation of Balb/c 3T3 cells. ERW was prepared by electrolysis of 0.002 M NaOH solution using a batch-type electrolysis device. Balb/c 3T3 cells were treated with 3-methyl cholanthrene (MCA) as an initiation substance, followed by treatment with phorbol-12-myristate-13-acetate (PMA) as a promotion substance. MCA/PMA-induced formation of a transformation focus was strongly suppressed by ERW supplemented with Pt nps but not by ERW or Pt nps individually. ERW supplemented with Pt nps suppressed transformation at the promoter stage, not at initiation, suggesting that **ERW supplemented with Pt nps suppressed the PMA-induced augmentation of intracellular ROS. ERW supplemented with Pt nps is a potential new antioxidant against carcinogenesis.**

PMID: 19003049 [PubMed - in process]

Int J Hyg Environ Health. 2005;208(6):481-8. Epub 2005 Oct 10.

Chlorinated river and lake water extract caused oxidative damage, DNA migration and cytotoxicity in human cells.

Yuan J, Wu XJ, Lu WQ, Cheng XL, Chen D, Li XY, Liu AL, Wu JJ, Xie H, Stahl T, Mersch-Sundermann V.
Department of Occupational and Environmental Health, Tongji Medical College of Huazhong University of Science and Technology, Wuhan, PR China.

Abstract
Consumption of chlorinated drinking water is suspected to be associated with adverse health effects, including mutations and cancer. In the present study, the genotoxic potential of water from Donghu lake, Yangtze river and Hanjiang river in Wuhan, an 8-million metropolis in China, was investigated using HepG2 cells and the alkaline version of the comet assay. It could be shown that all water extracts caused dose-dependent DNA migration in concentrations corresponding to dried extracts of 0.167-167 ml chlorinated drinking water per ml medium. To explore whether the intracellular redox status is regulated by chlorinated drinking water, we determined lipid peroxidation (LPO) and depletion of reduced glutathione (GSH). The malondialdehyde (thiobarbituric acid (TBA)-reactive aldehydes) concentration increased after chlorinated drinking water treatment of HepG2 cells in a dose-dependent manner, the GSH content decreased. The activity of lactate dehydrogenase (LDH) increased in chlorinated drinking water treated HepG2 cells indicating cytotoxicity. **In accordance with former studies which dealt with in vivo and in vitro micronucleus induction the present study shows that chlorinated drinking water from polluted raw water may entail genetic risks.**
PMID: 16325558 [PubMed - indexed for MEDLINE]

Life Science. 2006 Nov 10;79(24):2288-92. Epub 2006 Aug 2.

Anti-diabetic effects of electrolyzed reduced water in streptozotocin-induced and genetic diabetic mice.

Kim MJ, Kim HK. Department of Obesity management, Graduate School of Obesity Science, Dongduk Women's University, 23-1 Wolkgukdong, Seoul, 136-714, South Korea.

Oxidative stress is produced under diabetic conditions and is likely involved in progression of pancreatic beta-cell dysfunction found in diabetes. Both an increase in reactive oxygen free radical species (ROS) and a decrease in the antioxidant defense mechanism lead to the increase in oxidative stress in diabetes. Electrolyzed reduced water (ERW) with ROS scavenging ability may have a potential effect on diabetic animals, a model for high oxidative stress. Therefore, the present study examined the possible anti-diabetic effect of ERW in two different diabetic animal models. The genetically diabetic mouse strain C57BL/6J-db/db (db/db) and streptozotocin (STZ)-induced diabetic mouse were used as insulin deficient type 1 and insulin resistant type 2 animal model, respectively. ERW, provided as a drinking water, significantly reduced the blood glucose concentration and improved glucose tolerance in both animal models. However, ERW fail to affect blood insulin levels in STZ-diabetic mice whereas blood insulin level was markedly increased in genetically diabetic db/db mice. This improved blood glucose control could result from enhanced insulin sensitivity, as well as increased insulin release. The present data suggest that ERW may function as an orally effective anti-diabetic agent and merit further studies on its precise mechanism. PMID: 16945392

Biol Pharm Bull. 2007 Feb;30(2):234-6.

Preservative effect of electrolyzed reduced water on pancreatic beta-cell mass in diabetic db/db mice.

Kim MJ, Jung KH, Uhm YK, Leem KH, Kim HK.
Department of Obesity Management, Graduate School of Obesity Science, Dongduk Women's University, Seoul, South Korea.
mijakim@dongduck.ac.jp

Oxidative stress is produced under diabetic conditions and involved in progression of pancreatic beta-cell dysfunction. Both an increase in reactive oxygen free radical species (ROS) and a decrease in the antioxidant defense mechanism lead to the increase in oxidative stress in diabetes. Electrolyzed reduced water (ERW) with ROS scavenging ability may have a potential effect on diabetic animals, a model for high oxidative stress. Therefore, the present study examined the possible anti-diabetic effect of ERW in genetically diabetic mouse strain C57BL/6J-db/db (db/db). ERW with ROS scavenging ability reduced the blood glucose concentration, increased blood insulin level, improved glucose tolerance and preserved beta-cell mass in db/db mice. **The present data suggest that ERW may protect beta-cell damage and would be useful for anti-diabetic agent.**
PMID: 17268057 [PubMed - indexed for MEDLINE]

Biophys Chem. 2004 Jan 1;107(1):71-82.

The mechanism of the enhanced antioxidant effects against superoxide anion radicals of reduced water produced by electrolysis.

Hanaoka K, Sun D, Lawrence R, Kamitani Y, Fernandes G.

We reported that reduced water produced by electrolysis enhanced the antioxidant effects of proton donors such as ascorbic acid (AsA) in a previous paper. We also demonstrated that reduced water produced by electrolysis of 2 mM NaCl solutions did not show antioxidant effects by itself. We reasoned that the enhancement of antioxidant effects may be due to the increase of the ionic product of water as solvent. The ionic product of water (pKw) was estimated by measurements of pH and by a neutralization titration method. As an indicator of oxidative damage, Reactive Oxygen Species- (ROS) mediated DNA strand breaks were measured by the conversion of supercoiled phiX-174 RF I double-strand DNA to open and linear forms. **Reduced water had a tendency to suppress single-strand breakage of DNA induced by reactive oxygen species produced by H2O2/Cu (II) and HQ/Cu (II) systems.** The enhancement of superoxide anion radical dismutation activity can be explained by changes in the ionic product of water in the reduced water.

Biomed Res. 2009 Oct;30(5):263-9.

Electrolyzed-reduced water inhibits acute ethanol-induced hangovers in Sprague-Dawley rats.

Park SK, Qi XF, Song SB, Kim DH, Teng YC, Yoon YS, Kim KY, Li JH, Jin D, Lee KJ. Department of Environmental Medical Biology, Wonju College of Medicine, Yonsei University, Wonju, Gangwon, Republic of Korea.

Ethanol consumption disturbs the balance between the pro- and anti-oxidant systems of the organism, leading to oxidative stress. Electrolyzed-reduced water (ERW) is widely used by people in East Asia for drinking purposes because of its therapeutic properties including scavenging effect of reactive oxygen species. This study was performed to investigate the effect of ERW on acute ethanol-induced hangovers in Sprague-Dawley rats. Alcohol concentration in serum of ERW-treated rats showed significant difference at 1 h, 3 h and 5 h respectively as compared with the rats treated with distilled water. Both alcohol dehydrogenase type 1 and acetaldehyde dehydrogenase related with oxidation of alcohol were significantly increased in liver tissue while the level of aspartate aminotransferase and alanine aminotransferase in serum was markedly decreased 24 h after pre-oral administration of ERW. Moreover, oral administration of ERW significantly activated non-ezymatic (glutathione) and enzymatic (glutathione peroxidase, glutathione-S-transferase, Cu/Zn-superoxide dismutase and catalase) antioxidants in liver tissues compared with the control group. **These results suggest that drinking ERW has an effect of alcohol detoxification by antioxidant mechanism and has potentiality for relief of ethanol-induced hangover symptoms.** PMID: 19887722 [PubMed - in process]

Drug Dev Ind Pharm. 2009 Feb;35(2):145-53.

Effect of several electrolyzed waters on the skin permeation of lidocaine, benzoic Acid, and isosorbide mononitrate.

Kitamura T, Todo H, Sugibayashi K.
Faculty of Pharmaceutical Sciences, Josai University, Saitama, Japan.

Abstract
The effects of several electrolyzed waters were evaluated on the permeation of model base, acid and non-ionized compounds, lidocaine (LC), benzoic acid (BA), and isosorbide mononitrate (ISMN), respectively, through excised hairless rat skin. Strong alkaline-electrolyzed reducing water (ERW) enhanced and suppressed the skin permeation of LC and BA, respectively, and it also increased the skin permeation of ISMN, a non-ionized compound. On the contrary, strong acidic electrolyzed oxidizing water (EOW) enhanced BA permeation, whereas suppressing LC permeation. Only a marginal effect was observed on the skin permeation of ISMN by EOW. These marked enhancing effects of ERW on the skin permeation of LC and ISMN were explained by pH partition hypothesis as well as a decrease in skin impedance. **The present results strongly support that electrolyzed waters, ERW and EOW, can be used as a new vehicle in topical pharmaceuticals or cosmetics to modify the skin permeation of drugs without severe skin damage.**

81

J Food Sci. 2010 Mar;75(2):M111-5.

Combined effects of alkaline electrolyzed water and citric acid with mild heat to control microorganisms on cabbage.

Rahman SM, Jin YG, Oh DH.
Dept. of Food Science and Biotechnology and Inst. of Bioscience and Biotechnology, Kangwon Natl. Univ., Chuncheon, Gangwon 200-701, Republic of Korea.

Effects of alkaline electrolyzed water (AlEW), acidic electrolyzed water (AcEW), 100 ppm sodium hypochlorite (NaClO), deionized water (DIW), 1% citric acid (CA) alone, and combinations of AlEW with 1% CA (AlEW + CA), in reducing the populations of spoilage bacteria and foodborne pathogens on cabbage were investigated at various dipping times (3, 5, and 10 min) with different dipping temperatures (1, 20, 40, and 50 degrees C). Inhibitory effect of the selected optimal treatment against Listeria monocytogenes and Escherichia coli O157 : H7 on cabbage were also evaluated. Compared to the untreated control, **AlEW treatment most effectively reduced the numbers of total bacteria, yeast, and mold,** followed by AcEW and 100-ppm NaClO treatments. All treatments dip washed for 5 min significantly reduced the numbers of total bacteria, yeast, and mold on cabbage. With increasing dipping temperature from 1 to 50 degrees C, the reductions of total bacteria, yeast, and mold were significantly increased from 0.19 to 1.12 log CFU/g in the DIW wash treatment ($P < 0.05$). Combined 1% CA with AlEW treatment at 50 degrees C showed the reduction of around 3.98 and 3.45 log CFU/g on the total count, and yeast and mold, effective reduction of L. monocytogenes (3.99 log CFU/g), and E. coli O157 : H7 (4.19 log CFU/g) on cabbage. **The results suggest that combining AlEW with CA could be a possible method to control food-borne pathogens and spoilage bacteria effectively on produce.**

PMID: 20492239 [PubMed - in process

Artificial Organs, Volume 24, Issue 12, pages 984–987, December 2000

Effect of Electrolyzed Water on Wound Healing

Naoki Yahagi[1], Masashi Kono[1], Masaki Kitahara[1], Akito Ohmura[1], Osao Sumita[2], Toshimasa Hashimoto[3], Katsuaki Hori[3], Chen Ning-Juan[3], Paul Woodson[4], Shoji Kubota[5], Arata Murakami[6], Shinichi Takamoto[6]

Abstract

Electrolyzed water accelerated the healing of full-thickness cutaneous wounds in rats, but only anode chamber water (acid pH or neutralized) was effective. Hypochlorous acid (HOCl), also produced by electrolysis, was ineffective, suggesting that these types of electrolyzed water enhance wound healing by a mechanism unrelated to the well-known antibacterial action of HOCl. One possibility is that reactive oxygen species, shown to be electron spin resonance spectra present in anode chamber water, might trigger early wound healing through fibroblast migration and proliferation.

83

J Biosci Bioeng. 2010 Sep;110(3):308-13. Epub 2010 Apr 18.

In vitro inactivation of Escherichia coli, Staphylococcus aureus and Salmonella spp. using slightly acidic electrolyzed water.

Issa-Zacharia A, Kamitani Y, Tiisekwa A, Morita K, Iwasaki K.
Department of Environmental Science & Technology, Faculty of
Agriculture, Kagoshima University, 1-21-24 Korimoto, Kagoshima
890-0065, Japan.

Abstract

In the current study, the effectiveness of slightly acidic electrolyzed
water (SAEW) on an in vitro inactivation of Escherichia coli (E.
coli), Staphylococcus aureus (S. aureus) and Salmonella spp. was
evaluated and compared with other sanitizers. SAEW (pH 5.6,
23mg/l available chlorine concentration; ACC; and 940mV oxidation
reduction potential; ORP) was generated by electrolysis of dilute
solution of HCl (2%) in a chamber of a non-membrane electrolytic
cell. One milliliter of bacteria suspension (ca. 10-11 log(10)CFU/ml)
was mixed with 9ml of SAEW, strong acidic electrolyzed water
(StAEW; ca. 50mg/l ACC), sodium hypochlorite solution (NaOCl;
ca.120mg/l ACC) and distilled water (DW) as control and treated for
60s. SAEW effectively reduced the population of E. coli, S. aureus
and Salmonella spp. by 5.1, 4.8, and 5.2 log(10)CFU/ml. Although,
ACC of SAEW was more than 5 times lower than that of NaOCl
solution, they showed no significant bactericidal difference (p>0.05).
However, the bactericidal effect of StAEW was significantly higher
(p<0.05) than SAEW and NaOCl solution in all cases. When tested
with each individual test solution, E. coli, S. aureus and Salmonella
spp. reductions were not significantly different (p>0.05). These
findings indicate that SAEW with low available chlorine
concentration can equally inactivate E. coli, S. aureus and Salmonella
spp. as NaOCl solution and therefore **SAEW shows a high potential
of application in agriculture and food industry as an
environmentally friendly disinfection agent.**

J Food Prot. 2008 Sep;71(9):1934-47.

Electrolyzed water and its application in the food industry.

Hricova D, Stephan R, Zweifel C.
Institute for Food Safety and Hygiene, Vetsuisse Faculty University of Zurich, Winterthurerstrasse 272, 8057 Zurich, Switzerland.

Abstract

Electrolyzed water (EW) is gaining popularity as a sanitizer in the food industries of many countries. By electrolysis, a dilute sodium chloride solution dissociates into acidic electrolyzed water (AEW), which has a pH of 2 to 3, an oxidation-reduction potential of >1,100 mV, and an active chlorine content of 10 to 90 ppm, and basic electrolyzed water (BEW), which has a pH of 10 to 13 and an oxidation-reduction potential of -800 to -900 mV. Vegetative cells of various bacteria in suspension were generally reduced by > 6.0 log CFU/ml when AEW was used. However, AEW is a less effective bactericide on utensils, surfaces, and food products because of factors such as surface type and the presence of organic matter. Reductions of bacteria on surfaces and utensils or vegetables and fruits mainly ranged from about 2.0 to 6.0 or 1.0 to 3.5 orders of magnitude, respectively. Higher reductions were obtained for tomatoes. For chicken carcasses, pork, and fish, reductions ranged from about 0.8 to 3.0, 1.0 to 1.8, and 0.4 to 2.8 orders of magnitude, respectively. Considerable reductions were achieved with AEW on eggs. On some food commodities, treatment with BEW followed by AEW produced higher reductions than did treatment with AEW only. EW technology deserves consideration when discussing industrial sanitization of equipment and decontamination of food products. Nevertheless, decontamination treatments for food products always should be considered part of an integral food safety system. Such treatments cannot replace strict adherence to good manufacturing and hygiene practices.

85

Journal of the Internation Society of Sports Nutrition, 2010
September 13;7(1):29.

Acid-base balance and hydration status following consumption of
mineral-based alkaline bottled water. Heil DP.

ABSTRACT: BACKGROUND: **The present study sought to
determine whether the consumption of a mineral-rich alkalizing
bottled water could improve both acid-base balance and hydration
status in young healthy adults under free-living conditions.** The
mineral-rich alkalizing bottled water contains a naturally high mineral
content along with Alka-PlexLiquidTM, a dissolved supplement that
increases the mineral content and gives the water an alkalizing pH of
10.0. METHODS: Thirty-eight subjects were matched by gender and
self-reported physical activity (SRPA, hrs/week) and then split into
Control (12 women, 7 men; Mean+/-SD: 23+/-2 yrs; 7.2+/-3.6 hrs/week
SRPA) and Experimental (13 women, 6 men; 22+/-2 yrs; 6.4+/-4.0
hrs/week SRPA) groups. The Control group consumed non-mineralized
placebo bottled water over a 4-week period while the Experimental group
consumed the placebo water during the 1st and 4th weeks and the
mineral-rich alkalizing bottled water during the middle 2-week treatment
period. Fingertip blood and 24-hour urine samples were collected three
times each week for subsequent measures of blood and urine osmolality
and pH, as well as total urine volume. Dependent variables were analyzed
using multivariate repeated measures ANOVA with post-hoc focused on
evaluating changes over time within Control and Experimental groups
(alpha = 0.05). RESULTS: There were no significant changes in any of
the dependent variables for the Control group. The Experimental group,
however, showed significant increases in both the blood and urine pH
(6.23 to 7.07 and 7.52 to 7.69, respectively), a decreased blood and
increased urine osmolality, and a decreased urine output (2.51 to 2.05
L/day), all during the second week of the treatment period (P<0.05).
Further, these changes reversed for the Experimental group once subjects
switched to the placebo water during the 4th week. CONCLUSIONS:
**Consumption of mineral-rich alkalizing bottled water was associated
with improved acid-base balance (i.e., an alkalization of the blood
and urine) and hydration status when consumed under free-living
conditions. In contrast, subjects who consumed the placebo bottled
water showed no changes over the same period of time. These results
indicate that the habitual consumption of mineral-rich alkalizing
bottled water may be a valuable nutritional vector for influencing
both acid-base balance and hydration status in healthy adults.** PMID:
20836884

Food Chem Toxicol. 2009 Aug;47(8):2031-6. Epub 2009 May 27.

Hepatoprotective effect of electrolyzed reduced water against carbon tetrachloride-induced liver damage in mice.

Tsai CF, Hsu YW, Chen WK, Chang WH, Yen CC, Ho YC, Lu FJ.
Institute of Medicine, College of Medicine, Chung Shan Medical University, No. 110, Sec. 1, Jianguo N. Rd., Taichung 402, Taiwan.

The study investigated the protective effect of electrolyzed reduced water (ERW) against carbon tetrachloride (CCl(4))-induced liver damage. Male ICR mice were randomly divided into control, CCl(4), CCl(4)+silymarin, and CCl(4)+ERW groups. CCl(4)-induced liver lesions include leukocytes infiltration, hepatocyte necrosis, ballooning degeneration, mitosis, calcification, fibrosis and an increase of serum alanine aminotransferase (ALT), and aminotransferase (AST) activity. In addition, CCl(4) also significantly decreased the activities of superoxide dismutase (SOD) and glutathione peroxidase (GSH-Px). By contrast, ERW or silymarin supplement significantly ameliorated the CCl(4)-induced liver lesions, lowered the serum levels of hepatic enzyme markers (ALT and AST) and increased the activities of SOD, catalase, and GSH-Px in liver. **Therefore, the results of this study show that ERW can be proposed to protect the liver against CCl(4)-induced oxidative damage in mice, and the hepatoprotective effect might be correlated with its antioxidant and free radical scavenging effect.**

P M I D :   1 9 4 7 7 2 1 6

Biological & Pharmaceutical Bulletin. 2009 Feb;73(2):280-7. Epub 2009 Feb 7.

Enhanced induction of mitochondrial damage and apoptosis in human leukemia HL-60 cells due to electrolyzed-reduced water and glutathione.

Tsai CF, Hsu YW, Chen WK, Ho YC, Lu FJ. Institute of Medicine, Chung Shan Medical University, Taichung, Taiwan.

Electrolzyed-reduced water (ERW) is a higher pH and lower oxidation-reduction potential water. In the present study, we examined the enhanced effect of ERW in the apoptosis of leukemia cells (HL-60) induced by glutathione (GSH). An enhanced inhibitory effect on the viability of the HL-60 cells was observed after treatment with a combination of ERW with various concentrations of GSH, whereas no cytotoxic effect in normal peripheral blood mononuclear cells was observed. The results of apoptotic related protein indicated that the induction of HL-60 cell death was caused by the induction of apoptosis through upregulation of Bax and downregulation of Bcl-2. The results of further investigation showed a diminution of intracellular GSH levels in ERW, and combination with GSH groups. **These results suggest that ERW is an antioxidant, and that ERW, in combination with GSH, has an enhanced apoptosis-inducing effect on HL-60 cells, which might be mediated through the mitochondria-dependent pathway.**

PMID: 19202298

Biol Pharm Bull. 2011;34(11):1671-7.

Histological study on the effect of electrolyzed reduced water-bathing on UVB radiation-induced skin injury in hairless mice.

Yoon KS, Huang XZ, Yoon YS, Kim SK, Song SB, Chang BS, Kim DH, Lee KJ. Source Department of Environmental Medical Biology, Wonju College of Medicine, Yonsei University, Wonju, Gangwon, South Korea.

Abstract

Electrolyzed reduced water (ERW), functional water, has various beneficial effects via antioxidant mechanism in vivo and in vitro. However there is no study about beneficial effects of ERW bathing. This study aimed to determine the effect of ERW bathing on the UVB-induced skin injury in hairless mice. For this purpose, mice were irradiated with UVB to cause skin injury, followed by individually taken a bath in ERW (ERW-bathing) and tap water (TW-bathing) for 21 d. We examined cytokines profile in acute period, and histological and ultrastructural observation of skin in chronic period. We found that UVB-mediated skin injury of ERW-bathing group was significantly low compared to TW control group in the early stage of experiment. Consistently, epidermal thickening as well as the number of dermal mast cell was significantly lowered in ERW-bathing group. Defection of corneocytes under the scanning electron microscope was less observed in ERW-bathing group than in TW-bathing group. Further, the level of interleukin (IL)-1_, tumor necrosis factor (TNF)-_ and IL-12p70 in ERW group decreased whereas those of IL-10 increased. **Collectively, our data indicate that ERW-bathing significantly reduces UVB-induced skin damage through influencing pro-/anti-inflammatory cytokine balance in hairless mice. This suggests that ERW-bathing has a positive effect on acute UVB-mediated skin disorders. This is the first report on bathing effects of ERW in UVB-induced skin injury.**
PMID: 22040878 [PubMed - in process]

Food Microbiol. 2011 May;28(3):484-91. Epub 2010 Oct 27.

Combination treatment of alkaline electrolyzed water and citric acid with mild heat to ensure microbial safety, shelf-life and sensory quality of shredded carrots.

Rahman SM, Jin YG, Oh DH. Department of Food Science and Biotechnology, Institute of Bioscience and Biotechnology, Kangwon National University, Chuncheon, Gangwon 200-701, Republic of Korea.

Abstract
The objective of this study was to determine the synergistic effect of alkaline electrolyzed water and citric acid with mild heat against background and pathogenic microorganisms on carrots. Shredded carrots were inoculated with approximately 6-7 log CFU/g of Escherichia coli O157:H7 (932, and 933) and Listeria monocytogenes (ATCC 19116, and 19111) and then dip treated with alkaline electrolyzed water (AlEW), acidic electrolyzed water (AcEW), 100 ppm sodium hypochlorite (NaOCl), deionized water (DaIW), or 1% citric acid (CA) alone or with combinations of AlEW and 1% CA (AlEW + CA). The populations of spoilage bacteria on the carrots were investigated after various exposure times (1, 3, and 5 min) and treatment at different dipping temperatures (1, 20, 40, and 50 °C) and then optimal condition (3 min at 50 °C) was applied against foodborne pathogens on the carrots. When compared to the untreated control, treatment AcEW most effectively reduced the numbers of total bacteria, yeast and fungi, followed by AlEW and 100 ppm NaOCl. Exposure to all treatments for 3 min significantly reduced the numbers of total bacteria, yeast and fungi on the carrots. As the dipping temperature increased from 1 °C to 50 °C, the reductions of total bacteria, yeast and fungi increased significantly from 0.22 to 2.67 log CFU/g during the wash treatment ($p \leq 0.05$). The combined 1% citric acid and AlEW treatment at 50 °C showed a reduction of the total bacterial count and the yeast and fungi of around 3.7 log CFU/g, as well as effective reduction of L. monocytogenes (3.97 log CFU/g), and E. Coli O157:H7 (4 log CFU/g). **Combinations of alkaline electrolyzed water and citric acid better maintained the sensory and microbial quality of the fresh-cut carrots and enhanced the overall shelf-life of the produce.**

PMID: 21356455 [PubMed - indexed for MEDLINE]

Cytotechnology. 2011 Mar;63(2):119-31. Epub 2010 Nov 10

Suppressive effects of electrolyzed reduced water on alloxan-induced apoptosis and type 1 diabetes mellitus.

Li Y, Hamasaki T, Nakamichi N, Kashiwagi T, Komatsu T, Ye J, Teruya K, Abe M, Yan H, Kinjo T, Kabayama S, Kawamura M, Shirahata S. Department of Bioscience and Biotechnology, Faculty of Agriculture, Kyushu University, 6-10-1 Hakozaki, Higashi-ku, Fukuoka, 812-8581, Japan.

Abstract
Electrolyzed reduced water, which is capable of scavenging reactive oxygen species, is attracting recent attention because it has shown improved efficacy against several types of diseases including diabetes mellitus. Alloxan produces reactive oxygen species and causes type 1 diabetes mellitus in experimental animals by irreversible oxidative damage to insulin-producing _-cells. Here, we showed that electrolyzed reduced water prevented alloxan-induced DNA fragmentation and the production of cells in sub-G1 phase in HIT-T15 pancreatic _-cells. Blood glucose levels in alloxan-induced type 1 diabetes model mice were also significantly suppressed by feeding the mice with electrolyzed reduced water. **These results suggest that electrolyzed reduced water can prevent apoptosis of pancreatic _-cells and the development of symptoms in type 1 diabetes model mice by alleviating the alloxan-derived generation of reactive oxygen species.**
PMID: 21063772 [PubMed] PMCID: PMC3080478 [Available on 2012/3/1]

J Biosci Bioeng. 2010 Sep;110(3):308-13. Epub 2010 Apr 18.

In vitro inactivation of Escherichia coli, Staphylococcus aureus and Salmonella spp. using slightly acidic electrolyzed water.

Issa-Zacharia A, Kamitani Y, Tiisekwa A, Morita K, Iwasaki K.
Department of Environmental Science & Technology, Faculty of Agriculture, Kagoshima University, 1-21-24 Korimoto, Kagoshima 890-0065, Japan.

Abstract
In the current study, the effectiveness of slightly acidic electrolyzed water (SAEW) on an in vitro inactivation of Escherichia coli (E. coli), Staphylococcus aureus (S. aureus) and Salmonella spp. was evaluated and compared with other sanitizers. SAEW (pH 5.6, 23mg/l available chlorine concentration; ACC; and 940mV oxidation reduction potential; ORP) was generated by electrolysis of dilute solution of HCl (2%) in a chamber of a non-membrane electrolytic cell. One milliliter of bacteria suspension (ca. 10-11 log(10)CFU/ml) was mixed with 9ml of SAEW, strong acidic electrolyzed water (StAEW; ca. 50mg/l ACC), sodium hypochlorite solution (NaOCl; ca.120mg/l ACC) and distilled water (DW) as control and treated for 60s. SAEW effectively reduced the population of E. coli, S. aureus and Salmonella spp. by 5.1, 4.8, and 5.2 log(10)CFU/ml. Although, ACC of SAEW was more than 5 times lower than that of NaOCl solution, they showed no significant bactericidal difference (p>0.05). However, the bactericidal effect of StAEW was significantly higher (p<0.05) than SAEW and NaOCl solution in all cases. When tested with each individual test solution, E. coli, S. aureus and Salmonella spp. reductions were not significantly different (p>0.05). These findings indicate that SAEW with low available chlorine concentration can equally inactivate E. coli, S. aureus and Salmonella spp. as NaOCl solution and therefore **SAEW shows a high potential of application in agriculture and food industry as an environmentally friendly disinfection agent.**
PMID: 20547336 [PubMed - indexed for MEDLINE]

J Food Prot. 2009 Sep;72(9):1854-61.

Reduction of Escherichia coli O157:H7 on produce by use of electrolyzed water under simulated food service operation conditions.

Pangloli P, Hung YC, Beuchat LR, King CH, Zhao ZH. Department of Food Science and Technology, University of Georgia, 1109 Experiment Street, Griffin, Georgia 30223-1797, USA.

Abstract
Treatment of fresh fruits and vegetables with electrolyzed water (EW) has been shown to kill or reduce foodborne pathogens. We evaluated the efficacy of EW in killing Escherichia coli O157:H7 on iceberg lettuce, cabbage, lemons, and tomatoes by using washing and/or chilling treatments simulating those followed in some food service kitchens. Greatest reduction levels on lettuce were achieved by sequentially washing with 14-A (amperage) acidic EW (AcEW) for 15 or 30 s followed by chilling in 16-A AcEW for 15 min. This procedure reduced the pathogen by 2.8 and 3.0 log CFU per leaf, respectively, whereas washing and chilling with tap water reduced the pathogen by 1.9 and 2.4 log CFU per leaf. Washing cabbage leaves for 15 or 30 s with tap water or 14-A AcEW reduced the pathogen by 2.0 and 3.0 log CFU per leaf and 2.5 to 3.0 log CFU per leaf, respectively. The pathogen was reduced by 4.7 log CFU per lemon by washing with 14-A AcEW and 4.1 and 4.5 log CFU per lemon by washing with tap water for 15 or 30 s. A reduction of 5.3 log CFU per lemon was achieved by washing with 14-A alkaline EW for 15 s prior to washing with 14-A AcEW for 15 s. Washing tomatoes with tap water or 14-A AcEW for 15 s reduced the pathogen by 6.4 and 7.9 log CFU per tomato, respectively. **Application of AcEW using procedures mimicking food service operations should help minimize cross-contamination and reduce the risk of E. coli O157:H7 being present on produce at the time of consumption.**

PMID: 19777886 [PubMed - indexed for MEDLINE

Appl Biochem Biotechnol. 2006 Nov;135(2):133-44.

Electrolyzed-reduced water protects against oxidative damage to DNA, RNA, and protein.

Lee MY, Kim YK, Ryoo KK, Lee YB, Park EJ. Department of Genetic Engineering, Soonchunhyang University, Asan, Chungnam 336-600, Korea. miyoung@sch.ac.kr

Abstract

The generation of reactive oxygen species is thought to cause extensive oxidative damage to various biomolecules such as DNA, RNA, and protein. In this study, the preventive, suppressive, and protective effects of in vitro supplementation with electrolyzed-reduced water on H2O2-induced DNA damage in human lymphocytes were examined using a comet assay. Pretreatment, cotreatment, and posttreatment with electrolyzed-reduced water enhanced human lymphocyte resistance to the DNA strand breaks induced by H2O2 in vitro. Moreover, electrolyzed-reduced water was much more effective than diethylpyrocarbonate-treated water in preventing total RNA degradation at 4 and 25 degrees C. In addition, electrolyzed-reduced water completely prevented the oxidative cleavage of horseradish peroxidase, as determined using sodium dodecyl sulfate-polyacrylamide gels. **Enhancement of the antioxidant activity of ascorbic acid dissolved in electrolyzed-reduced water was about threefold that of ascorbic acid dissolved in non-electrolyzed deionized water, as measured by a xanthine-xanthine oxidase superoxide scavenging assay system, suggesting an inhibitory effect of electrolyzedreduced water on the oxidation of ascorbic acid.**

PMID: 17159237 [PubMed - indexed for MEDLINE]

J Microbiol. 2006 Aug;44(4):417-22.

Antibacterial effect of electrolyzed water on oral bacteria.

Lee SH, Choi BK. Department of Oral Microbiology and Immunology, School of Dentistry, Seoul National University, Seoul, Republic of Korea.

Abstract
This study investigated the antibacterial effect of electrolyzed water on oral bacteria both in vitro and in vivo. Tap water was electrolyzed in a water vessel using platinum cell technology. The electrolyzed tap water (called Puri-water) was put in contact with five major periodontopathogens or toothbrushes contaminated with these bacteria for 30 sec. In addition, Puri-water was used as a mouthwash for 30 sec in 16 subjects and the antibacterial effect on salivary bacteria was evaluated. Puri-water significantly reduced the growth of all periodontopathogens in culture and on toothbrushes, and that of aerobic and anaerobic bacteria in saliva, when compared to the effect of tap water. It also significantly reduced mutans streptococci growing on mitis salivarius-bacitracin agar. **Our results demonstrate that the electrolyzed tap water is effective as a mouthwash and for toothbrush disinfection.**
PMID: 16953177 [PubMed - indexed for MEDLINE]

Kidney Int. 2006 Jul;70(2):391-8. Epub 2006 Jun 7.

Electrolyzed-reduced water reduced hemodialysis-induced erythrocyte impairment in end-stage renal disease patients.

Huang KC, Yang CC, Hsu SP, Lee KT, Liu HW, Morisawa S, Otsubo K, Chien CT. Department of Family Medicine, National Taiwan University College of Medicine and National Taiwan University Hospital, Taipei, Taiwan.

Abstract
Chronic hemodialysis (HD) patients increase erythrocyte susceptibility to hemolysis and impair cell survival. We explored whether electrolyte-reduced water (ERW) could palliate HD-evoked erythrocyte impairment and anemia. Forty-three patients undergoing chronic HD were enrolled and received ERW administration for 6 month. We evaluated oxidative stress in blood and plasma, erythrocyte methemoglobin (metHb)/ferricyanide reductase activity, plasma metHb, and proinflammatory cytokines in the chronic HD patients without treatment (n=15) or with vitamin C (VC)- (n=15), vitamin E (VE)-coated dialyzer (n=15), or ERW treatment (n=15) during an HD course. The patients showed marked increases (15-fold) in blood reactive oxygen species, mostly H_2O_2, after HD without any treatment. HD resulted in decreased plasma VC, total antioxidant status, and erythrocyte metHb/ferricyanide reductase activity and increased erythrocyte levels of phosphatidylcholine hydroperoxide (PCOOH) and plasma metHb. Antioxidants treatment significantly palliated single HD course-induced oxidative stress, plasma and RBC PCOOH, and plasma metHb levels, and preserved erythrocyte metHb /ferricyanide reductase activity in an order VC>ERW>VE-coated dialyzer. However, ERW had no side effects of oxalate accumulation easily induced by VC. Six-month ERW treatment increased hematocrit and attenuated proinflammatory cytokines profile in the HD patients. **In conclusion, ERW treatment administration is effective in palliating HD-evoked oxidative stress, as indicated by lipid peroxidation, hemolysis, and overexpression of proinflammatory cytokines in HD patients.**
PMID: 16760903 [PubMed - indexed for MEDLINE]

J Food Prot. 2004 Jul;67(7):1377-83.

Effects of water source, dilution, storage, and bacterial and fecal loads on the efficacy of electrolyzed oxidizing water for the control of Escherichia coli O157:H7.

Stevenson SM, Cook SR, Bach SJ, McAllister TA. Agriculture and Agri-Food Canada Research Centre, Lethbridge, Alberta, Canada T1J 4B1.

Abstract
To evaluate the potential of using electrolyzed oxidizing (EO) water for controlling Escherichia coli O157:H7 in water for livestock, the effects of water source, electrolyte concentration, dilution, storage conditions, and bacterial or fecal load on the oxidative reduction potential (ORP) and bactericidal activity of EO water were investigated. Anode and combined (7:3 anode:cathode, vol/vol) EO waters reduced the pH and increased the ORP of deionized water, whereas cathode EO water increased pH and lowered ORP. Minimum concentrations (vol/vol) of anode and combined EO waters required to kill 10(4) CFU/ml planktonic suspensions of E. coli O157:H7 strain H4420 were 0.5 and 2.0%, respectively. Cathode EO water did not inhibit H4420 at concentrations up to 16% (vol/vol). Higher concentrations of anode or combined EO water were required to elevate the ORP of irrigation or chlorinated tap water compared with that of deionized water. Addition of feces to EO water products (0.5% anode or 2.0% combined, vol/vol) significantly reduced (P < 0.001) their ORP values to < 700 mv in all water types. A relationship between ORP and bactericidal activity of EO water was observed. The dilute EO waters retained the capacity to eliminate a 10(4) CFU/ml inoculation of E. coli O157:H7 H4420 for at least 70 h regardless of exposure to UV light or storage temperature (4 versus 24 degrees C). At 95 h and beyond, UV exposure reduced ORP, significantly more so (P < 0.05) in open than in closed containers. Bactericidal activity of EO products (anode or combined) was lost in samples in which ORP value had fallen to < or = 848 mV. When stored in the dark, the diluted EO waters retained an ORP of > 848 mv and bactericidal efficacy for at least 125 h; with refrigeration (4 degrees C), these conditions were retained for at least 180 h. Results suggest that EO water may be an effective means by which to control E. coli O157:H7 in livestock water with low organic matter content.
PMID: 15270489 [PubMed - indexed for MEDLINE]

Neuropsychopharmacology. 2009 Jan;34(2):501-8.

Consumption of molecular hydrogen prevents the stress-induced impairments in hippocampus-dependent learning tasks during chronic physical restraint in mice.

Nagata K, Nakashima-Kamimura N, Mikami T, Ohsawa I, Ohta S. Department of Biochemistry and Cell Biology, Institute of Development and Aging Sciences, Graduate School of Medicine, Nippon Medical School, Nakahara-ku, Kawasaki, Japan.

Abstract

We have reported that hydrogen (H(2)) acts as an efficient antioxidant by gaseous rapid diffusion. **When water saturated with hydrogen (hydrogen water) was placed into the stomach of a rat, hydrogen was detected at several microM level in blood.** Because hydrogen gas is unsuitable for continuous consumption, we investigated using mice whether drinking hydrogen water ad libitum, instead of inhaling hydrogen gas, prevents cognitive impairment by reducing oxidative stress. Chronic physical restraint stress to mice enhanced levels of oxidative stress markers, malondialdehyde and 4-hydroxy-2-nonenal, in the brain, and impaired learning and memory, as judged by three different methods: passive avoidance learning, object recognition task, and the Morris water maze. Consumption of hydrogen water ad libitum throughout the whole period suppressed the increase in the oxidative stress markers and prevented cognitive impairment, as judged by all three methods, whereas hydrogen water did not improve cognitive ability when no stress was provided. Neural proliferation in the dentate gyrus of the hippocampus was suppressed by restraint stress, as observed by 5-bromo-2'-deoxyuridine incorporation and Ki-67 immunostaining, proliferation markers. The consumption of hydrogen water ameliorated the reduced proliferation although the mechanistic link between the hydrogen-dependent changes in neurogenesis and cognitive impairments remains unclear. **Thus, continuous consumption of hydrogen water reduces oxidative stress in the brain, and prevents the stress-induced decline in learning and memory caused by chronic physical restraint. Hydrogen water may be applicable for preventive use in cognitive or other neuronal disorders.**

J Trauma. 2000 Sep;49(3):511-4.

Effectiveness of electrolyzed oxidized water irrigation in a burn-wound infection model.

Nakae H, Inaba H. Department of Emergency and Critical Care Medicine, Akita University School of Medicine, Japan.

OBJECTIVE:
The purpose of the study was to determine whether electrolyzed oxidized water (EOW) functions as a bactericide in burn injury with Pseudomonas aeruginosa infection in a rat burn-wound model.

METHODS:
Anesthetized Sprague-Dawley rats (n = 31) were subjected to third-degree burns to 30% of total body surface area. Two days after injury, all rats were infected with P. aeruginosa using 1 mL of a suspension containing 1 x 10(8) colony-forming units. Rats were assigned to one of three groups: no irrigation (group I), irrigation with physiologic saline (group II), or irrigation with EOW (group III). Blood culture, endotoxin levels, and survival rates were determined.

RESULTS:
Survival rate was significantly higher in group III than in groups I or II (p < 0.0001). Serum endotoxin levels on day 3 after infection in group III were significantly lower than the levels in group I (p < 0.01) and group II (p < 0.01). There were significant differences between the three groups in the culture of P. aeruginosa (p < 0.05).

CONCLUSION:
Irrigation and disinfection with EOW may become useful in preventing burn-wound sepsis

References

[1] Adv Colloid Interface Sci. 2006 Nov 23;127(1):19-27. Epub 2006 Sep 6. Surfaces and interfacial water: evidence that hydrophilic surfaces have long-range impact. Zheng JM, Chin WC, Khijniak E, Khijniak E Jr, Pollack GH

[2] Physiol Rev. 1998 Apr;78(2):547-81. The free radical theory of aging matures. Beckman KB, Ames BN. Department of Molecular and Cell Biology, University of California, Berkeley 94720-3202, USA.

[3] Ann. NY Acad. Sci.;686:28.), 1993. Radicals, hydrogen peroxide, peroxynitrate and peroxynitrite. Pryor WA, Stone K. Oxidants in cigarette smoke.

[4] Int J Environ Res Public Health. 2009 February; 6(2): 445–462. Published online 2009 February; Tobacco Smoke: Involvement of Reactive Oxygen Species and Stable Free Radicals in Mechanisms of Oxidative Damage, Carcinogenesis and Synergistic Effects of Other Respirable Particles. Athanasios Valavanidis, Thomais Vlachagianni, and Konstantinos Fiotakis.

[5] J Clin Endocrinol Metab 85. 2970-2973. 2000. Glucose challenge stimulates reactive oxygen species (ROS) generation by leucocytes. Mohanty P., Hamouda W., Garg R., Aljada A., Ghanim H., Dandona P.

[6] Am J Clin Nutr 80. 51-57.2004; Aljada A., Ghanim H., Mohanty P., Syed T., Bandyopadhyay A., Dandona P.: Glucose intake induces an increase in activator protein 1 and early growth response 1 binding activities, in the expression of tissue factor and matrix metalloproteinase in mononuclear cells, and in plasma tissue factor and matrix metalloproteinase concentrations.

[7] J Clin Endocrinol Metab 86. 355-362.2001. The suppressive effect of dietary restriction and weight loss in the obese on the generation of reactive oxygen species by leukocytes, lipid peroxidation, and protein carbonylation. Dandona P., Mohanty P., Ghanim H., Aljada A., Browne R., Hamouda W., Prabhala A., Afzal A., Garg R.

[8] Kidney Int. 39:9–26, 1991. Role of bone in regulation of systemic acid-base balance. Green J., Kleeman R.

[9] Am. J. Clin. Nutr. 59:1356–1361. 1994. Estimation of the renal net acid excretion by adults consuming diets containing variable amounts of protein. Remer T., Manz F.

[10] World J Gastrointest Pharmacol Ther. 2011 Jun 6;2(3):17-26. Proton pump inhibitor-associated pneumonia: Not a breath of fresh air after all? Fohl AL, Regal RE.

[11] Dig Dis. 2011;29(2):229-34. Epub 2011 Jul 5. Effects of environment and lifestyle on gastroesophageal reflux disease. Sonnenberg A. Source Portland VA Medical Center, Oregon Health & Science University, Portland, Oreg., USA

[12] Osteoporos Int 7:1. EFFO and NOF (1997) Who are candidates for prevention and treatment for osteoporosis?. Melton LJ, 3rd, Atkinson EJ, O'Connor

[13] J Bone Miner Res 13:1915, 1998. Bone density and fracture risk in men. MK, et al.

[14.] J Bone Miner Res 7:1005, 1992. Perspective. How many women have osteoporosis? Melton LJ, 3rd, Chrischilles EA, Cooper C, et al.

[15.] Osteoporos Int 11:669, 2000 Long-term risk of osteoporotic fracture in Malmo. Kanis JA, Johnell O, Oden A, et al.

[16] The China Study, by Colin Caldwell, BenBella Books, 2005.

[17] Adv Colloid Interface Sci. 2006 Nov 23;127(1):19-27. Epub 2006 Sep 6. Surfaces and interfacial water: evidence that hydrophilic surfaces have long-range impact. Zheng JM, Chin WC, Khijniak E, Khijniak E Jr, Pollack GH.
[18] The Water Puzzle and the Hexagonal Key, Mu Shik Jhon, Uplifting Press, Inc, 2004, page 47, adapted from Table 2.

[19] Cytotechnology. 2005 Jan;47(1-3):97-105. Electrolyzed Reduced Water Supplemented with Platinum Nanoparticles Suppresses Promotion of Two-stage Cell Transformation. Nishikawa R, Teruya K, Katakura Y, Osada K, Hamasaki T, Kashiwagi T, Komatsu T, Li Y, Ye J, Ichikawa A, Otsubo K, Morisawa S, Xu Q, Shirahata S.

[20] J Chem Phys. 2007 Dec 21;127(23):234504.
The vibrational spectra of protonated water clusters: a benchmark for self-consistent-charge density-functional tight binding. Yu H, Cui Q.

[21] J Colloid and Interface Sci. 1991; 147, 443. Study on the Properties of Water Clusters. JY Yu, MS Jhon

[22] National Tsing Hua University Report No. GMC 0203001 dated 28th March 2002